Concepts and Skills in Physical Assessment

MARY JANE SAUVÉ, R.N., M.S.

Assistant Professor of Nursing,
California State College, Sonoma,
Rohnert Park, California

ANGELA PECHERER, R.N., M.S.

Assistant Professor of Nursing Education,
Intercollegiate Center for Nursing Education,
Spokane, Washington

W. B. SAUNDERS COMPANY/Philadelphia/London/Toronto

W. B. Saunders Company: West Washington Square
Philadelphia, PA 19105

1 St. Anne's Road
Eastbourne, East Sussex BN21 3UN, England

1 Goldthorne Avenue
Toronto, Ontario M8Z 5T9, Canada

Library of Congress Cataloging in Publication Data

Sauvé, Mary Jane

Concepts and Skills in Physical Assessment

1. Physical diagnosis.   2. Nursing.   I. Pecherer, Angela, joint author.   II. Title.

RT42.S28   616.07'54   76-20120

ISBN   0-7216-7939-0

Concepts and Skills in Physical Assessment   ISBN 0-7216-7939-0

Last digit is the print number: 9   8   7   6   5   4   3   2

PREFACE

This text is the result of our "trial-and-error" efforts to incorporate the skills of history taking and physical examination into our curriculum. The teaching-learning theory of the Department of Nursing at California State College, Sonoma, regards the role of the teacher as that of a facilitator who provides the student with options and choices in learning experiences. It therefore seemed appropriate to utilize a self-instructional approach to this subject matter. The plethora of physical diagnosis texts on all levels and the increase in the availability of audiovisual materials on this subject led us to the decision to develop our units in a syllabus format. It is our intention to clearly delineate those behaviors which the nurse must demonstrate in order to perform a systematic client assessment rather than to develop another physical assessment text.

Concepts and Skills in Physical Assessment provides a unique approach to the study and practice of physical assessment. It contains specific guidelines for learning in the form of cognitive objectives and clinical objectives. These guidelines enable the student to identify and assimilate the cogent material presented in the various offerings. Performance guide cards provide a "step-by-step" outline of each examination procedure. While it may be possible for some individuals to use this text independently, it is intended to be used in conjunction with a planned program in an institutional setting or with the guidance of a preceptor.

We would like to express appreciation to our students and colleagues who have reviewed and critiqued one or more self-instructional units. Particularly, we would like to thank Dorothy Blake, R.N., M.S., F.N.P., Margaret Dombaugh, R.N., M.S., C.M.W., and Robert S. Wilkes, M.D.

Drawings for this text were prepared by Gerry Kleynenberg.

Our special thanks are offered to Ms. Kimiko Terry, our secretary, who endured, with patience and forbearance, the many revisions of this text.

MARY JANE SAUVÉ, R.N., M.S.
ANGELA PECHERER, R.N., M.S.

CONTENTS

SECTION II HEAD AND NECK

INTRODUCTION

DIRECTIONS TO THE STUDENT

This text consists of 23 self-instructional units which have been designed to guide you through the acquisition of knowledge and skills related to physical assessment. You are encouraged to proceed at your own rate and to choose learning activities which you feel are consistent with your own learning style.

To proceed with each unit, first complete the pre-test and then read the rationale, which presents an overview of the material you are to learn. Review the glossary of terms and use a medical dictionary to look up any terms which you cannot easily describe or define. This process is very important and will facilitate your learning of the unit content. Brief definitions can be written beside each term to help you familiarize yourself with them.

The cognitive objectives provide specific guidelines of what you are to learn. Read them carefully before proceeding to any learning activity. Since some learning activities are more complex than others, use the cognitive objectives to help you focus on the necessary material.

The learning activities have been annotated to help you make a selection if a choice is available to you. The learning activities are not all equal in scope and depth, and your instructor or preceptor may have a preference for one approach over another. Work with your selected activity until you are confident that you can demonstrate the behaviors outlined in the cognitive objectives.

Take the self-test. Use the self-test key to see how well you have learned the material in the unit. The key provides a rationale for each answer. Difficulty with the self-test indicates a need to re-examine the material in the unit.

With successful completion of the cognitive portion of the unit, you are now ready to proceed to the clinical component. The clinical component either is incorporated within the body of the unit or is presented after a series of units to provide continuity for the examination procedure. If you are completing a series of units, such as Units 7 through 11, review the clinical objectives in Unit 12 and the corresponding performance guide cards in Appendix II. If the clinical component is incorporated in the unit, proceed to the clinical objectives for guidelines of the skills you are to demonstrate.

After reviewing the clinical objectives, gather the equipment necessary for the examination and remove the appropriate performance guide cards from Appendix II. You are now ready to proceed with your first client examination. Follow the procedure for the examination listed on the performance guide cards and describe both normal and abnormal findings in the response sheets. Analyze your data and S.O.A.P. your findings. If you have difficulty, refer to the Examples of Problem-Oriented Charting in Appendix I.

Complete the three response sheets and arrange to demonstrate the examination skills to your instructor or preceptor. During this time you may also wish to discuss any difficulties you had in completing the response sheets.

SOURCES OF LEARNING ACTIVITIES

Articles and Reprints

American Heart Association, 44 East 23rd Street, New York, New York   10010
"Examination of the Heart – Auscultation" by James J. Leonard and Frank W. Kroetz, 1967.

American Journal of Nursing, 10 Columbus Circle, New York, New York   10019
Programmed Instruction
"Patient Assessment: Examination of the Abdomen," *74*:1679, P-16, Sept. 1974.
"Patient Assessment: Examination of the Ear," *75*:1–24, P-19, March 1975.
"Patient Assessment: Examination of the Eye, Part I," *74*:1–24, P-17, Nov. 1974.
"Patient Assessment: Examination of the Head and Neck," *75*:1–24, P-20, May 1975.
"Patient Assessment: Taking a Patient's History," *74*:293, P-14, Feb. 1974.

Clinical Symposium Reprints, CIBA Pharmaceutical Corporation, 556 Morris Avenue, Summit, New Jersey   07901
"Cataracts"
"Diseases of the Eye"
"Diseases and Surgery of the Nose"
"Otologic Diagnosis and Treatment of Deafness"
"Rheumatoid Arthritis"
"Scoliosis"
"White Lesions of the Mouth"

Miller and Fink Corporation, P.O. Box 1245, Darien, Connecticut   06820
"Breast Problems," *Nursing Update*, Vol. 6, No. 11, November 1975.
"Breast Problems," *Nursing Update*, Vol. 6, No. 12, December 1975.

A. H. Robins Co., Richmond, Virginia   23220
"G.I. Series: Physical Examination of the Abdomen," Sept. 1969.

Audiovisual Material

Bates, Barbara: J. B. Lippincott Company, Philadelphia, Pennsylvania   19105
Sound motion pictures
"The Abdomen"

    "The Head and Neck"
    "The Heart"
    "The Female Genitalia, Anus and Rectum"
    "The Male Genitalia, Anus and Rectum"
    "The Musculoskeletal System"
    "The Neurological Examination — Parts I and II"
    "The Peripheral Vascular System"
    "The Thorax"
    "Pressures and Pulses"

Blue-Hill Educational Systems, Inc., 52 S. Main Street, Spring Valley, New York 10977
Video Tape Cassettes
    "Part I — History Taking"
    "Part II — Integument"
    "Part III — Head"
    "Part IV — Eyes — Parts A and B"
    "Part V — Ears"
    "Part VI — Nose"
    "Part VII — Mouth and Throat"
    "Part VIII — Neck"
    "Part IX — Lymph Nodes"
    "Part X — Breasts"
    "Part XIA and B — Respiratory System"
    "Part XIIA — Cardiovascular System — Peripheral Circulation"
    "Part XIIB — Cardiovascular System — Heart"
    "Part XIIC — Cardiovascular System — Heart"
    "Part XIID — Cardiovascular System — Heart"
    "Part XIII — Abdomen"
    "Part XIV — Gynecologic Examination"
    "Part XV — Genitourologic Examination"
    "Part XVI — Musculoskeletal System"
    "Part XVII — The Neurological Examination"

Concept Media, 1500 Adams Avenue, Costa Mesa, California 92626
Filmstrips and tapes
    "Auscultation of Heart Sounds"
    "Physical Assessment: Heart and Lungs"

Eli Lilly and Company, 307 East McCarty, Indianapolis, Indiana 42606
16-mm films
    "Female Pelvic Examination"
    "Venereal Lesions in the Male"

Medical Electronic Educational Services, Inc., 29423 West Six Mile Road, Livonia, Michigan
48152
Filmstrips and tapes
    "Physical Diagnosis in Patient Assessment — History Taking"

Merck, Sharp and Dohme, Division of Merck and Company, Inc., West Point, Pennsylvania
19486
Audio tapes
    "Cardiac Auscultation" by Abe Ravin, 1968.

National Audiovisual Center (GSA), Washington, D.C. 20409
Slides and tapes
  "Ophthalmoscopy: Basic Self-Instruction for Medical Students"

OMNI, Ortho Pharmaceutical Corporation, Department of Educational Services, Raritan, New Jersey 08869
Slides, tapes, video tape cassettes
  "Breast Examination"
  "Pelvic Examination"
  "Teaching Breast Self-Examination"

Thiokol/Humetrics Corporation, 6374 Arizona Circle, Los Angeles, California 90045
Audio tapes
  "Heart Sounds: What They Teach Us" by Antonio C. deLeon, Jr., 1975.
  "The Chest: Its Signs and Sounds" by George Druger, 1974.

Westinghouse Learning Health Services, 100 Park Avenue, New York, New York 10017
Filmstrips and tapes
  "Examination of the Heart"
  "Examination of the Thorax and Lungs"

Books

Abbott Laboratories: *An Atlas of Some Pathological Conditions of the Eye, Ear and Throat.* Abbott Laboratories, North Chicago, 1957.

Bates, Barbara: *A Guide to Physical Examination.* J. B. Lippincott Co., Philadelphia, 1974.

DeGowin, E. L., and DeGowin, R. L.: *Bedside Diagnostic Examination*, 2nd ed. The Macmillan Co., New York, 1969.

DeJong, Russell, N., et al.: *Essentials of the Neurological Examination.* Smith Kline & French Laboratories, Philadelphia, 1974.

Delp, M. H. and Manning, R. T.: *Major's Physical Diagnosis*, 8th ed. W. B. Saunders Co., Philadelphia, 1975.

Fowkes, W. C., Jr., and Hunn, V. K.: *Clinical Assessment for the Nurse Practitioner.* The C. V. Mosby Co., St. Louis, 1973.

Frank, M. J., and Alvarez-Mena, S. C.: *Cardiovascular Physical Diagnosis.* Year Book Medical Publishers, Inc., Chicago, 1973.

Gillies, Dee Ann, and Alyn, Irene B.: *Patient Assessment and Management by the Nurse Practitioner.* W. B. Saunders Co., Philadelphia, 1976.

Judge, R. D., and Zuidema, G. D. (Eds.): *Methods of Clinical Examination: A Physiologic Approach*, 3rd ed. Little, Brown and Co., Boston, 1974.

Levene, G. M., and Calnan, D. C.: *Color Atlas of Dermatology.* Year Book Medical Publishers, Inc., Chicago, 1974.

OMNI: *Breast Examination.* Ortho Pharmaceutical Corp., Raritan, New Jersey, 1974.

Plum, F., and Posner, J. A.: *Diagnosis of Stupor and Coma*, 2nd ed. F. A. Davis Co., Philadelphia, 1972.

Prior, J. A., and Silberstein, J. S.: *Physical Diagnosis*, 4th ed. The C. V. Mosby Co., St. Louis, 1973.

Sana, J. M., and Judge, R. D. (Eds.): *Physical Appraisal Methods in Nursing Practice.* Little, Brown and Co., Boston, 1975.

Sherman, J. L. and Fields, Sylvia K.: *Guide to Patient Evaluation.* Medical Examination Publishing Co., Inc., Flushing, New York, 1974.

Models

OMNI: Ortho Pharmaceutical Corporation, Department of Educational Services, Raritan, New Jersey 08869.
    "Gynny" — Pelvic model

SECTION I

GENERAL SURVEY

Name_________________________________

Date_________________________________

PRE-TEST

UNIT 1

1. The advantage(s) of problem-oriented charting is that
   a) it systematizes the identification of client problems.
   b) it provides a mechanism for assessing the quality of health care.
   c) it provides better organization for client records.
   d) it contains a defined data base which is an advantage over traditional source-oriented records.
   e) it accomplishes all of the above.

2. Which of the following is not a part of the data base?
   a) health history
   b) laboratory examination
   c) physical examination
   d) problem list

3. A patient problem is defined as
   1. anything which the health provider perceives as interfering with the quality of life of the client.
   2. anything the client perceives as interfering with his or her quality of life.
   3. anything which requires diagnostic or management plans.
   4. any abnormality which can be systematically studied.
   a) 1 only is correct.
   b) 2 only is correct.
   c) 1 and 4 are correct.
   d) 2 and 3 are correct.

4. An analysis of a comprehensive data base should yield
   1. a list of the client's physical problems only.
   2. all the bio-psycho-social problems of a given client.
   3. discrepancies which need further investigation.
   4. a description of the client's life, particularly his/her ability to adjust to stress.
   a) 2 and 3 are correct.
   b) 1 only is correct.
   c) 1 and 3 are correct.
   d) 2, 3, and 4 are correct.

5. The problem list
   a) serves as an index or table of contents to the client's record.
   b) is always placed in the physician's section of the chart.
   c) contains a record of the physical examination.
   d) contains only active problems.

6. The four basic components of problem-oriented charting are
   1. health history.
   2. data base.

      3. S.O.A.P.
      4. initial plans.
      5. problem list.
      6. patient profile.
  a) 1, 3, 4 and 6 are correct.
  b) 2, 3, 4 and 5 are correct.
  c) 1, 4, 5 and 6 are correct.
  d) 2, 4, 5 and 6 are correct.

7. Which of the following would not be identified as an active client problem?
  a) anxiety reaction
  b) allergy to penicillin
  c) blindness
  d) history of pneumonia

8. The initial plans in problem-oriented charting are
      1. designed to resolve specific problems.
      2. organized in two sections — diagnostic and therapeutic.
      3. organized in three sections — diagnostic, therapeutic and patient education.
  a) 1 and 2 are correct.
  b) 1 and 3 are correct.

9. S.O.A.P. is
      1. the format used in problem-oriented progress notes.
      2. an outline utilized in developing the data base.
      3. an abbreviation for subjective data, objective data, assessment and plan.
      4. an abbreviation utilized to organize flow sheet information for certain conditions, such as ketoacidosis.
  a) 4 only is correct.
  b) 1 and 3 are correct.
  c) 3 only is correct.
  d) none of the above are correct.

Indicate whether the following statements are True (a) or False (b).

10. ______ The patient problems are derived from several categories, i.e., anatomical (hernia), symptomatic (pain), social (unemployed), risk factors (smokes 3 packs cigarettes/day).

11. ______ Subjective data include the client's observations, complaints and past history.

12. ______ The diagnostic component of the initial plan contains orders for specific drugs, including the exact dosage.

13. ______ Problems on the problem list are always listed as diagnoses.

14. ______ The focus of problem-oriented charting is on defining major medical and nursing problems.

15. ______ The A. in S.O.A.P. consists of the health provider's interpretation of the subjective and objective data.

Match the following data with the component of problem-oriented charting in which you would expect to see it displayed.

16. _______ "The medication has really helped the pain."

17. _______ #3 depression

18. _______ Baseline laboratory data

19. _______ Inferior myocardial infarction
D   — serial enxymes X 3
T   — bed rest, with commode privileges
Pt ed — explained cardiac monitoring

20. _______ Patient profile

a) Data base
b) Problem list
c) Initial plan
d) S.O.A.P.

Number 1
Problem-Oriented Charting

RATIONALE

This self-instructional unit is designed to introduce you to the concept of problem-oriented medical records. The unit focuses upon utilizing systematically collected data to identify client problems and to develop care plans and progress notes which correspond to the identified problems. At the end of this unit you will be able to demonstrate an understanding of problem-oriented medical records by developing a client problem list and initial care plan from a given data base and by utilizing additional data to develop progress notes.

GLOSSARY OF TERMS

Data base____

Initial plans____

P.O.M.R.____

Problem list____

Progress notes____

S.O.A.P.____

COGNITIVE OBJECTIVES

At the end of this unit you will demonstrate knowledge of problem-oriented charting by your ability to:

1. Explain the rationale behind the development of problem-oriented charting.

2. List and describe the components of the data base.

3. Define what constitutes a client problem.

4. Analyze a given data base.
    a. Generate a list of questions posed by the data.
    b. Identify problems or discrepancies.

5. Construct a list of client problems utilizing the following categories as guidelines:
   a. A proven diagnosis.
   b. A physiological problem.
   c. A sign, symptom or syndrome.
   d. An abnormal laboratory value.
   e. Operations.
   f. Allergies.
   g. Demographic data — risk factors.
   h. Social problems.
   i. Psychological problems.

6. Differentiate between active and inactive problems.

7. Recall the organization of the initial plan and describe each section.

8. Describe the format for problem-oriented progress notes.
   a. Explain the terms subjective, objective, assessment, plan.

LEARNING ACTIVITIES

The Learning Activities contain the information necessary for meeting the Cognitive Objectives. Select one and proceed to work with it until you have mastered the material. Use the Cognitive Objectives as a study guide. A Self-Test is provided so that you can check how much you have learned. If you have difficulty with the Self-Test, please review the material in the unit before proceeding to the Clinical Objectives.

Reading Activities

a) Gillies and Alyn: *Patient Assessment and Management*, "Recording Data and Planning Care." Although the information to meet the objectives is contained in this chapter, you may find it helpful to do some supplementary reading. Suggested readings would contain examples or illustrations of the recording method.

b) Judge and Zuidema: *Methods of Clinical Examination: A Physiologic Approach*, "The Problem-Oriented Medical Information System." This chapter provides a comprehensive overview of the problem-oriented method. The appendix at the end of the text contains examples of a problem list, data base, initial plans and progress notes.

c) Sherman and Fields: *Guide to Patient Evaluation*, "Problem Orientation." This chapter provides an introduction to the concept of problem-oriented charting. In Appendices I and II at the end of the text you will find examples of a problem list and data base.

Audiovisual Activities

a) Blue-Hill Educational System, Inc.: "Part I — History Taking." This 60-minute video tape cassette broadly covers elements of the health history. The lecturer then proceeds to show how the history, physical examination and laboratory tests compose the data base. Development of problem list, initial plan and progress notes is also covered but not in great detail.

Supplemental Activities

a) Sana and Judge: *Physical Appraisal Methods in Nursing Practice*, "Problem-Oriented Documentation of Nursing Care." This chapter briefly explains the concept of problem-oriented charting. It utilizes an example of this approach to demonstrate the nurse's contribution to the care of a patient in a hospital setting.

b) Delp and Manning: *Major's Physical Diagnosis*, "The Clinical Process," pp. 72–87. The discussion offers a brief overview of the basic concepts and an example of the forms utilized at the University of Kansas Medical Center to implement this approach to record keeping.

SELF-TEST

This Self-Test is for you. Use it to check how well you have mastered the material presented in this unit. The answers follow the test.

1. The four components of problem-oriented charting are

  a) _________________________   c) _________________________

  b) _________________________   d) _________________________

2. Problem-oriented charting was primarily developed to
  a) provide a focus for client problems.
  b) organize data collected by a variety of health care workers.
  c) overcome the difficulty in retrieving information from the traditional source-oriented medical record.
  d) standardize communication among health care providers.

3. Which of the following is not a component of the data base?
  a) baseline laboratory results
  b) physical examination findings
  c) health history
  d) prognosis

Indicate whether the following statements are True (a) or False (b).

4. _______ The data base may be problem-specific or comprehensive.

5. _______ A client problem is defined as a problem which requires diagnostic or therapeutic interventions or interferes with the quality of life as perceived by the health provider.

6. _______ An analysis of a comprehensive data base should lead to the identification of the bio-psycho-social problems of the client.

7. _______ The problem list is always located in the front of the record.

8. _______ Initial plans are written for each identified problem listed. Primarily they consist of plans for additional diagnostic studies.

9. _______ The objective data found in the progress notes include the client's observations and supporting laboratory data.

10. _______ The number assigned to a problem in the initial problem list changes when additional diagnostic information is obtained.

Client problems are derived from several different categories. Match the following:

	Problems		*Categories*

11. _______ Depression   a) Physiological problem
                                                     b) Symptom

12. _______ pH 7.32 Po_2 65   c) Abnormal laboratory value
                                                     d) Social problem

13. _______ Dyspnea   e) Psychological problem

14. _______ Congestive heart failure

15. _______ Unheated house

16. The three components of the initial plan are

a) ____

b) ____

c) ____

17. The format for progress notes includes the number and problem title and organizes the information utilizing S.O.A.P. What does S.O.A.P. stand for? Explain each term.

SELF-TEST KEY

1. The four components of problem-oriented charting are the (a) data base, (b) problem list, (c) initial plans and (d) progress notes.

2. (c) The impetus for the development of problem-oriented charting was the difficulty in retrieving information from the traditional source-oriented records and the lack of specificity in the data base. The problem-oriented record has changed the focus of records from medical and nursing problems to patient problems and has greatly systematized the organization of the record, thereby improving communication among health care providers.

3. (d) A prognosis is an assessment of the client's status and normally is found in the progress notes. A complete data base consists of a comprehensive health history (including a client profile), the physical examination findings and the results of initial laboratory tests.

4. (a) True. A problem-specific data base is constructed for specific problems, such as hypertension or diabetes mellitus; a comprehensive data base is utilized to identify all the client's problems.

5. (b) False. A client problem is defined as anything which requires either diagnostic or therapeutic plans or anything which the *client* perceives as interfering with his or her quality of life.

6. (a) True. A comprehensive data base should yield data which will enable the health provider to identify physical and psycho-social problems.

7. (a) True. The problem list is placed at the beginning of the medical record and serves as the table of contents or index.

8. (b) False. The initial plans and the plan found in the progress notes are organized into three sections: (1) diagnosis (an outline of further studies), (2) therapeutic, or treatment, plans and (3) client education.

9. (b) False. Objective data consist of physical examination findings and laboratory results. The client's complaints and observations are listed under subjective data.

10. (b) False. The number assigned to a problem in the problem list does not change even though the statement of the problem may change. As more information is gathered, some problems initially listed separately may turn out to be parts of a single problem. An example of this situation is shown on the following initial problem list:

#1 Jaundice 9/18/75 $\longrightarrow$ Laennec's cirrhosis

#2 Hepatomegaly 9/18/75 $\longrightarrow$ Laennec's cirrhosis

On 9/16/75 problems 1 and 2 were listed as "jaundice" and hepatomegaly." An arrow was placed after each problem to indicate that further resolution was necessary. The date 9/18/75 over each arrow indicates that these problems were resolved on that date as being due to Laennec's cirrhosis. From 9/16/75 to 9/18/75, problems 1 and 2 were referred to as "jaundice" and "hepatomegaly," but from 9/18/75 on, they will be followed by "Laennec's cirrhosis."

11. (e) Depression is categorized as a psychological problem.

12. (c) Both are abnormal laboratory values.

13. (b) Dyspnea is a symptom.

14. (a) Congestive heart failure is a physiological problem.

15. (d) An unheated house would be categorized as a social problem.

16. The three components of the initial plans are
    (a) Diagnostic — list of disorders which have been ruled out and plans for gathering more data.
    (b) Therapeutic — plans for drug therapy or other treatment.
    (c) Client education — information the client and family has been given and plans for including client input in future plans for health care.

17. S.O.A.P. is the abbreviation for subjective data, objective data, assessment and plans. *Subjective data* is information supplied by the client. It consists of patient observations, symptoms and past health history.

Objective data consists of information gleaned from the physical examination and laboratory tests.

Assessment is the health provider's interpretation of the subjective and objective data and the prognosis.

Plans include diagnostic, therapeutic and client education plans.

CLINICAL COMPONENT

Having completed the cognitive portion of this unit, you are now ready to proceed to the Clinical Objectives. The purpose of the Clinical Component is to familiarize you with the process of utilizing problem-oriented charting.

CLINICAL OBJECTIVES

At the end of this unit you will be able to develop a problem list from a given data base, develop initial plans for each identified problem and utilize S.O.A.P. in the formulation of progress notes. You will:

1. Demonstrate analysis of a given data base by constructing a client problem list which
   a. identifies physical and psycho-social problems.
   b. identifies problems that need further investigation.
   c. differentiates between active and inactive problems.

2. Devise initial plans for each identified problem from the data base.
   a. Diagnostic – plans for further studies.
   b. Therapeutic – medications and other forms of therapy.
   c. Client teaching – information given the patient and family.

3. Formulate progress notes
   a. utilizing a number and problem title for each.
   b. utilizing the S.O.A.P. format.

ACTIVITY

Utilizing the given data base which follows, practice constructing a problem list and an initial plan on Response Sheet 1. Response Sheets 2 and 3 will each provide a short data base and a problem title. Construct progress notes using the S.O.A.P. format. Refer to Appendix I for examples of a problem list, initial plans, and progress notes.

RESPONSE SHEET 1—PROBLEM-ORIENTED CHARTING

Client __Mrs. Mary Smith__

Date __3/17/76__   Age __79__   Sex __F__

Examiner __K. Jones, R.N.__

I. Informant

Mrs. Smith and daughter, Mrs. Lock.

II. Chief Complaint

Shortness of breath.

III. History of Present Illness

Mrs. Smith has noted episodes of squeezing substernal heaviness in her chest associated with marked dyspnea and frequent dizziness for past 3 months. She denies "real pain," fainting, nausea and diaphoresis. The episodes occur at rest as well as on exertion and have awakened her at night. The sensation usually lasts 10 min to 1 hr and abates spontaneously. Relief is gained at night by sitting up or walking around room. During past few months she has also noted pedal edema in the evenings and frequent nocturia (up 2X per night) but denies cough. She also thinks she has gained weight.

She has noted increasing fatigue and dyspnea on exertion over past several years which she attributes to old age. She is unable to complete one flight of stairs before stopping. She has slept on two pillows "for years." She has noted cramping in both calves occasionally on physical exertion but rarely at rest. The client also complains of severe constipation with rectal bleeding for one year — small amount of bright red blood in stool and on paper.

IV. Past Medical History (Include dates, severity, complications, if any)

A. Pediatric and Adult Illnesses

Mumps	Scarlet fever	Ulcer
(Measles) age 30	Tuberculosis	Jaundice
Chickenpox	Rheumatic fever	Renal disease
Pertussis	Arthritis	Rheumatism
Pneumonia	Diabetes mellitus	(Cystitis) age 62
Hepatitis	(Hypertension) age 63	VD
Rubella	Heart disease	Anemia

Comments: Cystitis, 1959, no sequelae. Neg. everything else. Hypertension diagnosed by previous physician who states he tried her on medication which she was "unable to tolerate." "It made me jumpy."

B. Immunizations

(Diphtheria) 1960	Polio	Mumps
(Tetanus) 1960	Measles	PPD
(Pertussis) 1960	Rubella	Other: Smallpox, 1918

C. Hospitalizations

Hysterectomy 28 yr ago (age 51)
Doesn't remember reason. No complications.

D. Injuries

None

E. Transfusions

None

F. Obstetrics

Grav i   Para i
Abortions: 0   Stillbirths: 0   Premature births: 0

G. Current Medications (Including contraceptive pills)

Vitamin C, 100 mg daily, "to keep down colds"
MOM, 1 or 2X/wk for constipation
No other medications

H. Allergies

Sulfa drugs

V. Family History

Age (L)	Age (D)	List parents, spouse, children, siblings	Health/Cause of death	TB	Diabetes	Glaucoma	Heart disease	Epilepsy	Alcoholism	Stroke	Hypertension	Obesity	Gout	Cancer	Jaundice	Kidney disease	Mental illness
	82/1942	Father	"Old age"			x											
	86/1950	Mother	"Old age"								x	x					
	82/1975	Husband	Myocardial infarction														
51		Daughter	Good									x					
82		Sister	Good	x							x						
	68/1963	Brother	Stroke				x			x							

VI. Social and Personal History

Birthplace: Cedar Rapids, Iowa   Date of birth: May 26, 1897   Education: 10th grade
Race: Caucasian
Residence(s):
    1897–1918 Cedar Rapids, Iowa
    1918 In France during WWI
    1919–1942 New York City
    1942–1970 San Francisco
    1970 to present: 112 Bennett Drive
                    Santa Rosa, CA
                    (daughter's home)

Occupations:
    Red Cross volunteer in WWI
    School teacher until married in 1924
    Housewife and mother
    1950–1962 – Salesperson in department store

Nature of present occupation (stresses, hazards, adaptation): Retired

Financial status:
    Social Security pension – $179/month
    Widow's pension – $200/month

Marital status: M   S   (W)   Sep   D   Number of children: 1
    Ages and sexes of children: 1 daughter, 51 yr old

Client's position in family: youngest of 3; great-grandmother

Religion: Lutheran

Military experience, foreign travel: France – 1918

Habits (tobacco, alcohol, nonprescription drugs, other): "Has never smoked." Wine – 4 oz @ bedtime. MOM 1 or 2X/wk. Vitamin C daily. ASA, gr X, for occasional headache, leg pain.

Diet (est. caloric intake, meal distribution, idiosyncrasies): Eats three meals per day. Est. caloric intake 1000 kcal/day. Has been anorexic last 3 wk. "Food doesn't seem to digest well."

Brief description of average day: Rise @ 7 am. Light breakfast – tea, toast, cereal. Cleans and straightens room, walks to store (three blocks). Lunch @ 12 noon. Watches TV or attends functions @ Senior Citizens Center (takes bus). Fixes dinner for working daughter and husband. Supper @ 6:30 pm. Retires by 10 pm. Bedroom on first floor.

VII. Review of Systems

Circle positive responses and explain below. Underline negative responses. If information not available, leave unmarked.

Genl	Wt loss	(Fatigue)	(Anorexia)	Night sweats	(Weakness)	Chills	Fever
Skin	Itch	Rash	Lesions	(Bruising) rt arm	Bleeding	Color change	

Eyes	<u>Pain</u>　　<u>Disch</u>　　<u>Itch</u>　　(Vision loss)　　<u>Diplopia</u>　　<u>Excessive tearing</u>
	(Glasses) / Contact lenses　　　　Date of last eye exam:　6/7/74
Ears	<u>Earaches</u>　　<u>Disch</u>　　<u>Tinnitus</u>　　(Hearing loss)
Nose	<u>Obstruction</u>　　<u>Disch</u>　　<u>Epistaxis</u>
Throat & Mouth	<u>Sore throats</u>　　<u>Bleeding gums</u>　　(Toothache)　　(Dentures) full, since 1960
Neck	<u>Swelling</u>　　<u>Dysphagia</u>　　<u>Hoarseness</u>
Chest	<u>Cough</u>　　<u>Sputum</u>: amt & characteristics　　<u>Hemoptysis</u>　　<u>Wheeze</u>
	Freq URI's　　Pain on resp　　(Dyspnea)
	Breasts:　<u>Lumps</u>　　Pain　　Bleeding　　Disch
CV	<u>Precordial pain</u>　　<u>Palpitation</u>　　(Dyspnea on exertion)
	(Paroxysmal nocturnal dyspnea)　　(Orthopnea)　　(Edema)　　Heart murmur
	Thrombophlebitis　　(Claudication)
GI	(Heartburn)　　<u>Nausea</u>　　<u>Vomit</u>　　<u>Diarrhea</u>　　<u>Food intolerance</u>
	(Excessive gas or indigestion)　　(Constipation)　　Change in BM　　<u>Jaundice</u>
	Bloating　　Melena　　Hemorrhoids　　<u>Hernia</u>　　<u>Pain</u>　　(Rectal bleeding)
GU	<u>Dysuria</u>　　Freq　　(Nocturia)　　<u>Retention</u>　　<u>Polyuria</u>　　(Dribbling)
	<u>Hematuria</u>　　<u>Flank pain</u>　　Disch　　Infections
	Male:　Penile disch　　Lesion　　Hx of VD　　Testicular pain　　Mass
	Infertility　　Impotence　　Libido
	Female:　Menarche at age:　14　　Last menstrual period:　1948
	Flow　　Days　　Menopause　　Abnormal bleeding
Extrem	<u>Joint pains</u>　　<u>Varicose veins</u>　　(Claudication) occ　　<u>Back pain</u>　　(Edema)
	(Stiffness)　　<u>Deformities</u>
Endo	<u>Hot flashes</u>　　<u>Hair loss</u>　　Temp intolerance　　Polydipsia　　Goiter
Neurol	<u>Numbness</u>　　<u>Tingling</u>　　<u>Tremor</u>　　Fainting　　Headaches
	<u>Muscle weakness</u>　　Ataxia　　<u>Paralysis/Paresis</u>　　(Dizziness)　　Seizures

	Memory loss	Unconsciousness		
Psych	Anxiety	Depression	Insomnia	Sexual problems	Therapy
	Nightmares			
Other				

VIII. Client Profile (Summarize in narrative form your impressions of the client)

A pleasant, moderately obese 79-yr-old-widow, retired and presently living with her married daughter. She has her own room on the first floor of a two-story house. She is receiving both Social Security and pension benefits. She states she "has a comfortable income" that allows her to help with groceries and also stay active in church and social clubs. Mrs. Smith seems to be well adjusted and mentally alert. She describes herself as active and involved. She expresses concern about her present condition as it is interfering with her normal activities and her plans to visit her great-grandchildren.

Physical examination:
   Vital signs: Pulse 85 irreg. Resp. 12 unlabored. Temp. 98°F, oral
   Blood pressure: Supine   R arm 160/90   L arm 160/100
      Sitting   R arm 164/92
      Standing R arm 162/90
   Weight: 130 lb
   Height: 60 inches
   General: Pale, moderately obese 79-yr-old female in no apparent distress.
   Integument: Good turgor — skin very dry, scaly on forearms and legs, ecchymosis on right upper arm, nails brittle but in good repair. Hair distribution normal.
   Lymph nodes: Nonpalpable.
   Skull: Normocephalic. No bruits or discomfort.
   Eyes: Lacrimal ducts open, cornea clear and convex, sclera white, conjunctiva clear. PERRLA. Visual field intact, ocular movement normal. Red reflex normal. Fundi — cup/disc ratio 1:2; arterioles narrowed; AV ratio 3:5, AV nicking both fundi. Linear hemorrhage. OS 1 DO away at 2 o'clock.
   Ears: Pinna normal configuration — no tophi, no discharge. TM's clear, no perforations. Light reflex present. Can hear whisper 2″ from ear. Air conduction > bone conduction, *no* lateralization.
   Mouth, nose and throat: Sinuses nontender to palpation. Membranes pink — upper and lower dentures, tonsils scarred. Gag reflex present.
   Neck: Full ROM. Trachea midline, thyroid not palpable. Veins distended 3 cm above clavicle — fill from below.
   Breasts: Symmetrical. Contour and consistency appropriate to age. No retractions, nipple discharge, masses or tenderness.
   Thorax: Respiratory rate: 12 normal excursion. Respiratory rhythm: regular, unlabored. Chest wall: slight kyphosis, expansion equal bilaterally. Slight increase in AP diameter. No tenderness. Tactile fremitus normal throughout. Equal diaphragmatic excursion. Resonant percussion note over all lung fields. Normal breath sounds except for a few fine basilar rales which did not clear with cough.
   Cardiovascular system: External jugular veins are distended 3 cm above clavicle @ 45° elevation. Prominent A wave. No HJR. Apical impulse evident at 5th intercostal space 14 cm LSB. No epigastric pulsations noted. PMI as above diameter 3 cm, slow, sustained impulse. No heave, thrill or rib retraction. S_1 louder than S_2 at apex. S_3 also present in supine and left lateral position. Rate 92 irreg. Pulse deficit. $A_2 > P_2$. No murmurs or rubs.

Popliteal and pedal pulses decreased both lower extremities. Carotid, femoral, brachial and radial pulses normal. Bruits over left carotid and both femorals. Calves tender to touch, neg. for Homans' sign. No purpura, inflammation or varicosities. Feet cooler than legs with fair capillary pulse. No cyanosis, clubbing or splinter hemorrhages.

Abdomen: Soft, nontender, slightly distended. No skin lesions, pulsations or hernia noted. Bowel sounds normal. Liver edge in costal margin, nontender.

Genitalia: Normal distribution of pubic hair, no labial swelling or lesions. Normal clitoris. Introitus admits two fingers. No urethral redness or discharge. Vaginal mucus dry, red. Discharge — pink, serous 1+, no odor. Pap omitted. Rectal: Spinchter tone good. No external and internal hemorrhoids. Stool, brown, blood-flecked.

Joints: Good ROM in all joints. No deformity or tenderness. 1+ edema in both ankles. Slight kyphosis.

Neurological: Cerebral function. Alert, awake. Mental status: Intact, oriented to time, place, person. Cranial nerves: I not tested. II, vision 20/30, both eyes with glasses. II through XII, see ENT exam.

Cerebellar function. Gait normal. Finger-to-nose, heel-to-shin coordination intact. Romberg negative.

Motor system: No weakness or tremors. Muscle mass appropriate for age.

Sensory system: Intact to touch, vibration and pinprick.

Reflexes:

	Biceps	Triceps	Brachial	Knee	Achilles	Plantar
R	+ +	+ +	+ +	+ +	+ +	↓
L	+ +	+ +	+ +	+ +	+ +	↓

0 = absent	tr = trace	1+ = decreased
2+ = normal	3+ = hyperactive	4+ = sustained clonus

Laboratory data:
Hematology: WBC   11,000
  Hb   10 gm   Hct   38%
Chemistry: Na^+ 135 mEq/L   Blood sugar   96 mg%
  K^+ 4.5   BUN   18 mg%
  CO_2 20.00
  Cl   102
Urinalysis: Normal

Chest x-ray: Routine. Moderate cardiomegaly with some pulmonary vascular congestion bilaterally.
ECG: Atrial fibrillation with VR @ 96.

Student_______________________________________

Date_______________________________________

RESPONSE SHEET 1—PROBLEM-ORIENTED CHARTING

Client Problem List

Date Problem Entered	Active	Inactive

Student_________________________________

Date___________________________________

RESPONSE SHEET 2—PROBLEM-ORIENTED CHARTING

Data Base

Mr. D is a 66-yr-old man whose chief complaint is chest pain. He says the pain in his left side began about 24 hr ago and has been getting worse. The pain is constant and becomes knifelike when he coughs or moves suddenly. He is most comfortable sitting quietly or lying on his left side. He denies smoking or drinking, but states he has had a cough which produced a small amount of yellow sputum for the past 4 days. Prior to his present illness he states he was well and working full time. He has no history of previous chest pain or shortness of breath.

Physical examination revealed a well-nourished male who appeared physically younger than his age. Vital signs: blood pressure 145/80, pulse 104, respirations 22, oral temperature 100.4°F; no jugular distention was noted. Eyes, ears, nose, throat and neck were unremarkable. His chest was slightly tender laterally on the left side, and increased tactile fremitus was noted. Percussion note was decreased over the left lower lobe. Auscultation was normal except over the lower left lobe where medium rales were audible. His cardiovascular examination was normal. A chest x-ray revealed a left lower lobe infiltrate involving most of the lobe.

Progress Notes

Problem: Chest pain, fever, cough.

S. (Client's observations, complaints, health history)

O. (Physical findings)

A. (Assessment of the problem, data, prognosis)

P. (Plans for further evaluation, care, teaching)

RESPONSE SHEET 3—PROBLEM-ORIENTED CHARTING

Data Base

Mrs. R is a 30-yr-old woman whose chief complaint is vaginal bleeding. She is well developed, white, married, grav iii, para iii. Her menses began at age 12; are regular at intervals of about 30–32 days; lasting 4 days. She denies fever or chills. Two months ago she had an intrauterine device inserted. Since that time menses has occurred every 25–28 days and has lasted 7–9 days with copious flow. She has had abdominal cramping with each menses since IUD insertion. She is presently in the 6th day of menses.

Vital signs: blood pressure 110/70, pulse 100, respirations 18. Her abdomen is nontender, and external genitalia are normal. Episiotomy scar midline. Vaginal mucosa is intact and pink. The uterus is slightly tender, posterior, of average size and regular shape. The cervix is pink, compatible with multiparity and has a trickle of blood from the os. The adnexa are within normal limits. Rectal examination is negative.

Progress Notes

Problem: Vaginal bleeding

    S. (Client's observations, complaints, health history)

    O. (Physical findings)

    A. (Assessment of the problem, data, prognosis)

    P. (Plans for further evaluation, care, teaching)

PRE-TEST

UNIT 2

1. Open-ended dialogue is characterized by
   a) direct questioning techniques.
   b) indirect questions which encourage the client to freely express all concerns.
   c) questions which clarify details or focus the client on specific issues.
   d) questions which generate client responses which confirm your suspicions about the client's problem.

2. Which of the following represents an appropriate recording of a client's reason for seeking health care?
   a) Angina pectoris, duration 2 hr
   b) Substernal pain radiating to left axilla, 1 hr duration
   c) "Grabbing" chest pain, 2 days' duration
   d) Pleurisy, 2 days' duration

3. This 36-yr-old female is divorced and the sole support of her three children, ages 12, 9 and 5. She has a demanding position with an advertising agency which requires occasional out-of-town travel. She ingests an average of 20 oz of alcohol per week. She has not smoked for 5 years but reports smoking a pack of cigarettes per day for 10 years previously. This information constitutes elements found in the
   a) social/personal history.
   b) past health history.
   c) systems review.
   d) family history.

4. The purpose of the systems review includes
   1. gathering data about the past and present status of each body system.
   2. searching for symptoms which relate to the present client problem but may have been overlooked.
   3. gathering data concerning the client's chief problem.
   4. identifying problems that the client considers unimportant but may affect his future health status.
   a) 1 only is correct.
   b) 1, 2 and 4 are correct.
   c) 3 and 4 are correct.
   d) all of the above are correct.

5. In seeking a description of a symptom, the health professional should ascertain the
   1. location — what areas of the body are involved? If there is pain, does it radiate?
   2. type — how does the client describe it?
   3. duration — how long has it been present? If periodic, how long does each episode last?
   4. influencing factors — what aggravates or relieves the symptom?
   5. severity — mild or severe?
   a) 1, 2 and 3 are correct.
   b) 1, 2, 3 and 5 are correct.

      c) 3 and 5 are correct.
      d) all of the above are correct.

Match the following areas of the health history with the client statements in items 6 through 11.

      a) Chief complaint
      b) Present illness
      c) Past history
      d) Personal or social history
      e) Family history
      f) Review of systems

6. ______ "It started about 3 months ago. Each time I walk to the store I have to stop to relieve the pain. Lately I can only walk a block before the pain begins."

7. ______ "My mother died at 56 of cirrhosis. My father is 60 now and as far as I know in good health."

8. ______ "I had all my shots before going over to Nam in 1970."

9. ______ "I've been passing black stools all this week."

10. ______ "Yes, I have to get up every night to go to the bathroom. Sometimes twice. No, I don't have any pain or trouble starting my stream."

11. ______ "I was born in Pennsylvania. Worked in the coal mines 'til I finished school."

12. The primary goals of the health interview are to
    1. gather data to substantiate physical findings.
    2. establish rapport between the client and health care provider.
    3. obtain data about an individual's medical and emotional status.
    4. develop a complete data base for diagnosis.
    a) 4 only is correct.
    b) 2 and 3 are correct.
    c) 1 and 2 are correct.
    d) all of the above are correct.

13. Examples of nonverbal communication include
    a) body position.
    b) wringing of hands.
    c) refusal to maintain eye contact.
    d) all of the above.

14. Direct questioning is appropriate while gathering data
    a) for the review of systems.
    b) about the present illness.
    c) in the past medical history.
    d) in a and b.
    e) in none of the above.

15. An analysis of the client's personal/social history will enable the health professional to identify

1. genetic predispositions to illness.
2. support systems the client utilizes or that are available in his environment.
3. the client's health teaching needs.
4. the relationship of childhood diseases to present symptoms, if any.
5. the client's strengths and weaknesses, ability to meet basic needs and relationships within the family structure.

a) 1, 3 and 4 are correct.
b) 2, 4 and 5 are correct.
c) 2, 3 and 5 are correct.
d) all of the above are correct.

Indicate whether the following statements are True (a) or False (b).

16. _______ Verbal and nonverbal mannerisms which convey approval or disapproval can influence the type of information shared by the patient.

17. _______ Client behaviors during the interview may provide many clues about his feelings. It is important for the health professional to validate impressions of these feelings with the client.

18. _______ If a school health physical is the specific reason for an individual's seeking health care, it is recorded as the chief complaint.

19. _______ Collection of a complete health history is mandatory before any interventions are initiated with the client.

20. _______ Data concerning medically important and previously diagnosed illnesses are gathered during the client's narrative of past health problems.

Number 2
The Health History

RATIONALE

This self-instructional unit is designed to introduce you to the process of obtaining a health history. The unit focuses upon the components of the health history and presents an overview of interviewing techniques. At the end of this unit you will be able to demonstrate beginning facility in gathering a data base which will include an individual's current and past health problems, family health problems and relationships and activities within his environment.

GLOSSARY OF TERMS

Review the following terms before and after completing this unit. You should be able to define or describe them readily.

Chief complaint____

Diagnosis____

Direct questioning____

Nonverbal communication____

Open-ended questioning____

Psychological problem____

Risk factor____

Sign____

Social problem____

Symptom____

Syndrome____

COGNITIVE OBJECTIVES

At the end of this unit you will demonstrate knowledge of basic interviewing techniques and the components of the health history by your ability to:

1. Discuss the goals of the health interview.

2. Recognize and relate at least three behaviors which are essential to the establishment of an effective professional/client relationship.

3. Differentiate between direct and open-ended questioning and apply both forms to the various elements of the health history.

4. Define nonverbal communication. Give examples of nonverbal communication expressed by the client and health professional.

5. Recall and define the elements of the health history:
    a. Chief complaint.
    b. Present illness.
    c. Past history.
    d. Family history.
    e. Personal or social history.
    f. Review of systems.

6. Explain the importance of determining the factor(s) which influenced the individual to seek health care.
    a. The major health problem, if any, and its duration.
    b. The type of examination – school health physical, periodic check-up, evaluation of acute or chronic illness.

7. Dissect an individual's narrative about the present illness into onset, chronology of events and current status.

8. Identify and list data which illustrate components of an individual's past medical history.

9. Outline the type of data used to develop a personal or social profile of the individual.

10. Describe the importance of obtaining a family history.

11. Explain the rationale for a systems review.

LEARNING ACTIVITIES

The Learning Activities contain the information necessary for meeting the Cognitive Objectives. Select one and proceed to work with it until you have mastered the material. Use the Cognitive Objectives as a study guide. A Self-Test is provided so that you can check how much you know. If you have difficulty with the Self-Test, please review the material in this unit.

Reading Activities

a) Delp and Manning: *Major's Physical Diagnosis*, "The Clinical Process," sensitively discusses the components of the client/professional relationship. The chapter provides a very brief overview of interview principles and adequately covers material on elements of health history.

b) Gillies and Alyn: *Patient Assessment and Management by the Nurse Practitioner*, "Techniques of Health Interviewing" and "The Content of the Patient's Medical History." These two chapters present a fairly comprehensive summary of the interviewing process with several illustrative samples of questioning techniques. The components of the health history are cogently described and illustrated.

c) Prior and Silberstein: *Physical Diagnosis*, "Medical History." The chapter briefly describes components of client/professional relationship and principles of interviewing. It utilizes an interesting, very readable format in presenting elements of health history.

d) Sherman and Fields: *Guide to Patient Evaluation*, "The Process of Interviewing" and "Health History I and II." A brief overview of the principles of interviewing is followed by a discussion of the elements of the health history. The authors have divided the health history into two parts: the initial interview which lends itself to open-ended questioning and the collection of background data which lends itself to more direct questioning.

Audiovisual Activities

a) Blue-Hill Educational Systems, Inc.: "Part I – History Taking." This 60-minute video tape cassette begins with a general introduction to the process of history taking. It broadly covers elements of health history and its relationship to the assessment of the client. Interviewing techniques are not covered.

Supplemental Activities

a) Frances Mechner: "Taking a Patient's History — A Programmed Unit," in *AJN*, February 1974, p. 293.

b) Medical Electronic Educational Services, Inc.: "Physical Diagnosis in Patient Assessment — History Taking." This audiotape-filmstrip presentation includes description of chief complaint, present illness and systems review.

c) Sana and Judge: *Physical Appraisal Methods in Nursing Practice*, "Nurse-Patient Communication and Relationship in the Physical Appraisal Process." Aspects of client/professional relationships and interviewing principles are discussed. This is an excellent review of concept of anxiety and its effect on communication and client behaviors.

SELF-TEST

This Self-Test is for you. Use it to check how well you have learned the material presented in the unit. The answers follow the test.

1. Which of the following *is not* a goal of the health interview?
   a) To acquire data concerning the client's present and past state of health
   b) To establish a working relationship between the client and health professional
   c) To provide additional learning experiences for the student.
   d) To provide support for clients and increase their understanding of health and illness

2. Which of the following behaviors displayed by the health professional is essential in establishing and maintaining an effective rapport with the client?

    a) Neat, clean appearance
    b) Listening to the client in a caring, unbiased, unhurried manner
    c) Utilizing the same format in every interview situation
    d) Conducting all interviews in absolute privacy

3. "Tell me about what you're usually doing when you notice the pain?" is an example of (open-ended/direct) questioning.

4. A client who begins to increase the distance between himself and the health professional during the interview may be demonstrating

    a) a wish to change the subject.
    b) a desire to conclude the interview.
    c) discomfort with the questioning.
    d) all of the above.

Match the following components of the health history with the data in items 5 through 10.

    a) Chief complaint
    b) Present illness
    c) Past health history
    d) Personal or social history
    e) Family history
    f) Review of systems

5. _______ Tonsillectomy, 1948. Pneumonia, 1960.

6. _______ Mother died, 1965. CVA age 65.

7. _______ "My knee began to swell 2 days ago and now I can hardly walk."

8. _______ Appetite, dietary habits, bowel habits, indigestion, flatus, vomiting, diarrhea, abdominal pain.

9. _______ "The pain started about 3 weeks ago but it seems to go away when I eat something."

10. _______ "I usually smoke a pack of cigarettes a day."

11. The health history of a client who is in obvious pain
    a) can be obtained later from a relative or friend.
    b) can be delayed until the client has been made as comfortable as possible in the situation.
    c) should be postponed until the client has been heavily medicated.
    d) should never be delayed.

12. Pain is a frequent complaint of individuals seeking medical help. List the five characteristics of pain which will enable you to gather information about the client's

present illness.

a) _______________________________   d) _______________________________

b) _______________________________   e) _______________________________

c) _______________________________

13. A review of the client's illnesses, surgery, medications, and injuries may provide valuable background data which may shed light on the current complaint. This information is primarily collected during
    a) the systems review.
    b) the history of present illness.
    c) the family history.
    d) the past health history.

14. Which of the following data should be included in the social/personal history?
    a) personality factors
    b) habits such as smoking, alcohol ingestion, sleep patterns
    c) possible exposure to tropical diseases and occupational hazards
    d) all of the above

15. The purpose of a systems review is
    a) to make a thorough evaluation of the client's past and present health status.
    b) to prevent omission of important data that may have been overlooked by the client or the health professional.
    c) to achieve the goals in both a and b.
    d) not given in the above choices.

SELF-TEST KEY

1. (c) While the medical interview will indeed provide the student with an additional learning experience, the primary purpose of the interview is to establish a working relationship which allows the reciprocal exchange of information between the client and the health professional.

2. (b) Clients enter the health care system because they are concerned about a problem which is affecting them. Therefore, the health professional who demonstrates an open, caring attitude, who reserves judgments on client statements and who allows the patient to tell his story in his own way will be successful in gaining the trust and cooperation of the client.

3. Open-ended. A question which elicits a maximum number of words from the client per minute and a minimum from the practitioner is considered open-ended. It is designed to obtain as many details as possible about the client's complaint.

4. (d) Clients who begin to shift back in their chairs or turn their heads from the practitioner are exhibiting signs of nonverbal communication which may indicate discomfort or a desire to avoid discussing the subject at hand.

5. (c) The recounting of past medical or surgical problems constitutes two of the elements to be collected during a review of the client's past medical history.

6. (e) Heredity and other constitutional factors play a role in the cause of certain diseases. Inquiry as to the current health status of the client's family, their ages if living, and if deceased the age at death and cause of death may be significant in the analysis of the client's complaint.

7. (a) This statement reflects the chief complaint or reason the individual is seeking medical intervention. It is recorded in the patient's own words as briefly as possible.

8. (f) During the systems review the client is asked questions regarding the past and present health state of each of the body systems. The data given in this example would elicit questions regarding the gastrointestinal tract.

9. (b) This response is an example of the type of information a client may give during the narrative of a present illness. It is important for the health professional to ascertain when the pain first began, the frequency of occurrence and any changes in symptoms which may have occurred during that interval of onset and the present time.

10. (d) Information regarding the client's habits, occupation and work history, sexual habits and responses to the stresses of daily living is acquired during the personal and social history.

11. (b) Client interviews should be held shortly after his entrance into the health care setting. However, if the client is in severe pain or very anxious, the interview can be postponed until such problems have been handled.

12. Type, location, duration, severity and factors which influence or precipitate pain are critical features of pain which should be explored with the client.

13. (d) A detailed review of the past health history of the individual may reveal that the symptoms are the sequelae of a previous acute illness.

14. (d) The client's emotional reactions, both to the medical problem and to the environment, will greatly influence the course of any health care intervention. Therefore, careful questioning directed toward gathering data regarding the client's habits, life, adjustments, occupation and personal interests will enhance the ability of the health professional to understand the client and make appropriate further plans.

15. (c) The goals of the systems review are (1) to evaluate as completely as possible the current and past health status of each organ system and (2) to prevent important clues from being overlooked by either the client or the health professional.

CLINICAL COMPONENT

Having completed the cognitive portion of this unit, you are now ready to proceed to the Clinical Objectives. The purpose of the Clinical Component is to enable you to utilize interviewing and assessment techniques to complete a health history, develop a client profile and initiate a problem list.

CLINICAL OBJECTIVES

At the end of this unit you will develop a client profile and initiate a partial problem list through an analysis of data collected during a health history. You will be able to:

1. Demonstrate application of interviewing techniques by
   a. providing a quiet, comfortable, private setting for the interview.
   b. initiating the interview with a clarification of your role, status and the purpose of the interaction.
   c. projecting an interested, understanding, unhurried attitude during the client's narrative.
   d. utilizing vocabulary which the client understands.
   e. utilizing both open-ended and direct questions to collect client data.
   f. listening carefully and nonjudgmentally to the client's story.

2. Demonstrate knowledge of the elements of the health history by
   a. briefly recording the chief complaint, utilizing the client's own words when possible.
   b. dissecting the client's narrative about the present illness into its critical components:
      1) Onset.
      2) Chronology of events.
      3) Current status.
      4) Reasons for seeking health care at present.
   c. completing a review of the client's past health problems, including
      1) diagnosed illnesses.
      2) surgical procedures.
      3) medications – past and current.
      4) injuries.
      5) gynecological and obstetrical data.
      6) allergies.
      7) immunizations.
   d. identifying health patterns within the client's family through a tabulation of
      1) the current age and health status of family members.
      2) the age at death and cause of death of other family members and relatives.
      3) the occurrence of specific disease entities within the family.
   e. eliciting risk factors from an account of the client's habits, educational and occupational history, geographical exposure, hobbies and marital or sexual history.
   f. reviewing past and current client symptoms experienced in each body system.

3. Demonstrate analysis of client data by
   a. constructing a client profile which includes
      1) birthplace, family position, religious affiliation and attitudes, education, residences and occupational background.
      2) marital status.
      3) nature of current occupation, stresses, hazards, adjustments.
      4) socioeconomic status.
      5) personality type and reactions to environment.
      6) daily routine and habits.
   b. systematically listing all the health problems suggested by the client's health history.

ACTIVITY

Utilizing three of your peers or clients in the clinical area, practice interviewing techniques by completing the following health history form. Remove the Performance Guide cards for Unit 2 located in Appendix II at the end of this book. These cards will enable you to practice the skills necessary to meet the Clinical Objectives and complete the Response Sheets. On each Response Sheet you will be expected to (1) ask questions which elicit possible symptoms, (2) systematically record client responses and (3) construct a client profile and initiate a partial problem list.

When you have mastered the Clinical Objectives and completed the Response Sheets, arrange to demonstrate your skills to your laboratory instructor or preceptor.

RESPONSE SHEET—HEALTH HISTORY

Client_______________________________

Date_______________________Age________Sex______

Examiner_______________________________

I. Informant

II. Chief Complaint

III. History of Present Illness

IV. Past Medical History (Include dates, severity, complications, if any)

    A. Pediatric and Adult Illnesses

Mumps	Scarlet fever	Ulcer
Measles	Tuberculosis	Jaundice
Chickenpox	Rheumatic fever	Renal disease
Pertussis	Arthritis	Rheumatism
Pneumonia	Diabetes mellitus	Cystitis
Hepatitis	Hypertension	VD
Rubella	Heart disease	Anemia
Other:		

    B. Immunizations

Diphtheria	Polio	Mumps
Tetanus	Measles	PPD
Pertussis	Rubella	Other:

C. Hospitalizations

D. Injuries

E. Transfusions

F. Obstetrics

Grav________Para_______

Abortions_______Stillbirths_______Premature births_______

G. Current Medications (Including contraceptive pills)

H. Allergies

V. Family History

Age		List parents spouse, children, siblings	Health/Cause of death	TB	Diabetes	Glaucoma	Heart disease	Epilepsy	Alcoholism	Stroke	Hypertension	Obesity	Gout	Cancer	Jaundice	Kidney disease	Mental illness	Other:
L	D																	
		Father																
		Mother																

VI. Social and Personal History

Birthplace: Education: Race:

Residence(s):

Occupation(s):

Nature of present occupation (stresses, hazards, adaptation):

Financial status:

Marital status: M   S   W   Sep   D   Number of children:

Ages and sexes of children:

Client's position in family:

Religion:

Military experience, foreign travel:

Habits (tobacco, alcohol, nonprescription drugs, other):

Diet (est. caloric intake, meal distribution, idiosyncrasies):

Brief description of average day:

VII. Review of Systems

Circle positive response and explain below. Underline negative response. If information not available, leave unmarked.

Genl	Wt loss Fatigue Anorexia Night sweats Weakness
	Chills Fever
Skin	Itch Rash Lesions Bruising Bleeding Color change
Eyes	Pain Disch Itch Vision loss Diplopia
	Excessive tearing Glasses/Contact lenses Date of last eye exam:
Ears	Earaches Disch Tinnitus Hearing loss
Nose	Obstruction Disch Epistaxis
Throat & Mouth	Sore throats Bleeding gums Toothache Dentures
Neck	Swelling Dysphagia Hoarseness
Chest	Cough Sputum: amt & char Hemoptysis Wheeze
	Freq URI's Pain on resp Dyspnea
	Breasts: Lumps Pain Bleeding Disch
CV	Precordial pain Palpitation Dyspnea on exertion
	Paroxysmal nocturnal dyspnea Orthopnea Edema
	Heart murmur Thrombophlebitis Claudication
GI	Heartburn Nausea Vomit Diarrhea Food intolerance
	Excessive gas or indigestion Constipation Change in BM
	Jaundice Bloating Melena Hemorrhoids Hernia
	Pain Rectal bleeding
GU	Dysuria Freq Nocturia Retention Polyuria
	Dribbling Hematuria Flank pain Disch Infections
	Male: Penile disch Lesion Hx of VD Testicular pain

	Mass Infertility Impotence Libido
	Female: Menarche at age: Last menstrual period:
	Flow Days Menopause Abnormal bleeding
Extrem	Joint pains Varicose veins Claudication Back pain
	Edema Stiffness Deformities
Endo	Hot flashes Hair loss Temp intolerance Polydipsia
	Goiter
Neurol	Numbness Tingling Tremor Fainting Headaches
	Muscle weakness Ataxia Paralysis/Paresis Dizziness
	Seizures Memory loss Unconsciousness
Psych	Anxiety Depression Insomnia Sexual problems
	Therapy Nightmares
Other	

VIII. Client Profile

Summarize in narrative form your impression of the client.

IX. Client Partial Problem List

Date Problem Entered	Active	Inactive
Date Problem Entered		

RESPONSE SHEET—HEALTH HISTORY

Client_______________________________

Date_______________________Age_______ Sex_______

Examiner_____________________________

I. Informant

II. Chief Complaint

III. History of Present Illness

IV. Past Medical History (Include dates, severity, complications, if any)

A. Pediatric and Adult Illnesses

Mumps	Scarlet fever	Ulcer
Measles	Tuberculosis	Jaundice
Chickenpox	Rheumatic fever	Renal disease
Pertussis	Arthritis	Rheumatism
Pneumonia	Diabetes mellitus	Cystitis
Hepatitis	Hypertension	VD
Rubella	Heart disease	Anemia
Other:		

B. Immunizations

Diphtheria	Polio	Mumps
Tetanus	Measles	PPD
Pertussis	Rubella	Other:

C. Hospitalizations

D. Injuries

E. Transfusions

F. Obstetrics

Grav_______Para_______

Abortions_______Stillbirths_______Premature births_______

G. Current Medications (Including contraceptive pills)

H. Allergies

V. Family History

Age		List parents spouse, children, siblings	Health/Cause of death	TB	Diabetes	Glaucoma	Heart disease	Epilepsy	Alcoholism	Stroke	Hypertension	Obesity	Gout	Cancer	Jaundice	Kidney disease	Mental illness	Other:
L	D																	
		Father																
		Mother																

VI. Social and Personal History

Birthplace: Education: Race:

Residence(s):

Occupation(s):

Nature of present occupation (stresses, hazards, adaptation):

Financial status:

Marital status: M   S   W   Sep   D   Number of children:

Ages and sexes of children:

Client's position in family:

Religion:

Military experience, foreign travel:

Habits (tobacco, alcohol, nonprescription drugs, other):

Diet (est. caloric intake, meal distribution, idiosyncrasies):

Brief description of average day:

VII. Review of Systems

Circle positive response and explain below. Underline negative response. If information not available, leave unmarked.

Genl	Wt loss Fatigue Anorexia Night sweats Weakness
	Chills Fever
Skin	Itch Rash Lesions Bruising Bleeding Color change
Eyes	Pain Disch Itch Vision loss Diplopia
	Excessive tearing Glasses/Contact lenses Date of last eye exam:
Ears	Earaches Disch Tinnitus Hearing loss
Nose	Obstruction Disch Epistaxis
Throat & Mouth	Sore throats Bleeding gums Toothache Dentures
Neck	Swelling Dysphagia Hoarseness
Chest	Cough Sputum: amt & char Hemoptysis Wheeze
	Freq URI's Pain on resp Dyspnea
	Breasts: Lumps Pain Bleeding Disch
CV	Precordial pain Palpitation Dyspnea on exertion
	Paroxysmal nocturnal dyspnea Orthopnea Edema
	Heart murmur Thrombophlebitis Claudication
GI	Heartburn Nausea Vomit Diarrhea Food intolerance
	Excessive gas or indigestion Constipation Change in BM
	Jaundice Bloating Melena Hemorrhoids Hernia
	Pain Rectal bleeding
GU	Dysuria Freq Nocturia Retention Polyuria
	Dribbling Hematuria Flank pain Disch Infections
	Male: Penile disch Lesion Hx of VD Testicular pain

	Mass Infertility Impotence Libido			
	Female: Menarche at age: Last menstrual period:			
	Flow Days Menopause Abnormal bleeding			
Extrem	Joint pains Varicose veins Claudication Back pain			
	Edema Stiffness Deformities			
Endo	Hot flashes Hair loss Temp intolerance Polydipsia			
	Goiter			
Neurol	Numbness Tingling Tremor Fainting Headaches			
	Muscle weakness Ataxia Paralysis/Paresis Dizziness			
	Seizures Memory loss Unconsciousness			
Psych	Anxiety Depression Insomnia Sexual problems			
	Therapy Nightmares			
Other				

VIII. Client Profile

Summarize in narrative form your impression of the client.

IX. Client Partial Problem List

Date Problem Entered	Active	Inactive

RESPONSE SHEET—HEALTH HISTORY

Client______________________________

Date________________Age______Sex______

Examiner____________________________

I. Informant

II. Chief Complaint

III. History of Present Illness

IV. Past Medical History (Include dates, severity, complications, if any)

A. Pediatric and Adult Illnesses

Mumps	Scarlet fever	Ulcer
Measles	Tuberculosis	Jaundice
Chickenpox	Rheumatic fever	Renal disease
Pertussis	Arthritis	Rheumatism
Pneumonia	Diabetes mellitus	Cystitis
Hepatitis	Hypertension	VD
Rubella	Heart disease	Anemia
Other:		

B. Immunizations

Diphtheria	Polio	Mumps
Tetanus	Measles	PPD
Pertussis	Rubella	Other:

C. Hospitalizations

D. Injuries

E. Transfusions

F. Obstetrics

Grav________Para________

Abortions________Stillbirths________Premature births________

G. Current Medications (Including contraceptive pills)

H. Allergies

V. Family History

Age		List parents spouse, children, siblings	Health/Cause of death	TB	Diabetes	Glaucoma	Heart disease	Epilepsy	Alcoholism	Stroke	Hypertension	Obesity	Gout	Cancer	Jaundice	Kidney disease	Mental illness	Other:
L	D																	
		Father																
		Mother																

VI. Social and Personal History

Birthplace: Education: Race:

Residence(s):

Occupation(s):

Nature of present occupation (stresses, hazards, adaptation):

Financial status:

Marital status: M   S   W   Sep   D   Number of children:

Ages and sexes of children:

Client's position in family:

Religion:

Military experience, foreign travel:

Habits (tobacco, alcohol, nonprescription drugs, other):

Diet (est. caloric intake, meal distribution, idiosyncrasies):

Brief description of average day:

VII. Review of Systems

Circle positive response and explain below. Underline negative response. If information not available, leave unmarked.

Genl	Wt loss Fatigue Anorexia Night sweats Weakness
	Chills Fever
Skin	Itch Rash Lesions Bruising Bleeding Color change
Eyes	Pain Disch Itch Vision loss Diplopia
	Excessive tearing Glasses/Contact lenses Date of last eye exam:
Ears	Earaches Disch Tinnitus Hearing loss
Nose	Obstruction Disch Epistaxis
Throat & Mouth	Sore throats Bleeding gums Toothache Dentures
Neck	Swelling Dysphagia Hoarseness
Chest	Cough Sputum: amt & char Hemoptysis Wheeze
	Freq URI's Pain on resp Dyspnea
	Breasts: Lumps Pain Bleeding Disch
CV	Precordial pain Palpitation Dyspnea on exertion
	Paroxysmal nocturnal dyspnea Orthopnea Edema
	Heart murmur Thrombophlebitis Claudication
GI	Heartburn Nausea Vomit Diarrhea Food intolerance
	Excessive gas or indigestion Constipation Change in BM
	Jaundice Bloating Melena Hemorrhoids Hernia
	Pain Rectal bleeding
GU	Dysuria Freq Nocturia Retention Polyuria
	Dribbling Hematuria Flank pain Disch Infections
	Male: Penile disch Lesion Hx of VD Testicular pain

	Mass Infertility Impotence Libido
	Female: Menarche at age: Last menstrual period:
	Flow Days Menopause Abnormal bleeding
Extrem	Joint pains Varicose veins Claudication Back pain
	Edema Stiffness Deformities
Endo	Hot flashes Hair loss Temp intolerance Polydipsia
	Goiter
Neurol	Numbness Tingling Tremor Fainting Headaches
	Muscle weakness Ataxia Paralysis/Paresis Dizziness
	Seizures Memory loss Unconsciousness
Psych	Anxiety Depression Insomnia Sexual problems
	Therapy Nightmares
Other	

VIII. Client Profile

Summarize in narrative form your impression of the client.

IX. Client Partial Problem List

Date Problem Entered	Active	Inactive
Date Problem Entered	Active	Inactive

PRE-TEST

UNIT 3

1. Skin lesions are evaluated for
    1. chronology.
    2. associated pain and pruritus.
    3. type, grouping and distribution.
    4. related causative factors.
    5. treatment modalities employed.
    a) 3 only is correct.
    b) 2 and 4 are correct.
    c) 2, 3 and 5 are correct.
    d) all of the above are correct.

Match each of the structures in items 2 through 5 with the appropriate function or description.

2. _______ Sebaceous gland
3. _______ Apocrine gland
4. _______ Dermis
5. _______ Eccrine gland

a) Sweat production for thermal regulation
b) Modified sweat gland which secretes waste products that cause body odors
c) Contains hair follicles, sweat glands and fat
d) Produces a fatty substance for lubrication and protection of the skin and hair
e) Contains blood vessels, connective tissue and sebaceous glands

6. A client with an abnormally pale complexion may have
    a) hyperpigmentation.
    b) large amounts of reduced hemoglobin in the blood.
    c) increased visibility of oxygenated hemoglobin in the blood.
    d) a low level of bilirubin in the blood.
    e) none of the above conditions.

Match each of the lesions in items 7 through 10 with its description.

7. _______ Macule
8. _______ Scale
9. _______ Papule
10. _______ Vesicle

a) Raised, solid mass, up to 0.05 cm in diameter
b) Fluid-filled skin elevation, up to 0.05 cm in diameter
c) Dried residue of blood, pus or serum
d) Thin flakes of epidermis
e) Nonelevated, well-circumscribed lesion, up to 1 cm in diameter

11. An area of thin, shiny skin with decreased visibility of normal skin markings is called
    a) lichenification.
    b) plaque.
    c) atrophy.
    d) keloid.

12. Conditions in which alopecia can occur include
    1. aging.
    2. hypothyroidism.
    3. fever.
    4. heavy metal poisoning.
  a) 1 and 3 are correct.
  b) 2 and 4 are correct.
  c) 1, 3 and 4 are correct.
  d) all of the above are correct.

13. The distribution of lesions found with a contact dermatitis would be described as
  a) symmetrical.
  b) localized.
  c) generalized.
  d) none of the above terms.

14. The configuration for lesions arranged in groups is described as
  a) annular.
  b) generalized.
  c) linear.
  d) clustered.

15. Examples of hemorrhagic lesions include
    1. purpura.
    2. petechiae.
    3. spider angiomas.
    4. lipomas.
    5. erosions.
  a) 1 and 2 are correct.
  b) 3 only is correct.
  c) 1 and 4 are correct.
  d) 2, 3 and 5 are correct.
  e) none of the above are correct.

16. Flattening of the angle between the nail and its base is
    1. found in subacute bacterial endocarditis.
    2. a description of spoon-shaped nails.
    3. related to calcium deficiency.
    4. described as clubbing.
    5. associated with chronic hypoxia.
  a) 1 and 2 are correct.
  b) 4 and 5 are correct.
  c) 2 and 3 are correct.
  d) 4 only is correct.

17. Elasticity and/or mobility of the skin is decreased by
    1. atrophy of the skin.
    2. systemic edema.
    3. intracellular dehydration.
    4. rapid loss of body tissue in dieting or malnutrition.
  a) 3 only is correct.
  b) 1 and 2 are correct.
  c) 1, 3 and 4 are correct.

  d) 2 only is correct.
  e) all of the above are correct.

18. Increased amounts of reduced hemoglobin circulating in the blood usually give light

   skin a _______________ appearance.
   a) bronze
   b) flushed
   c) bluish
   d) pale

19. Secondary lesions
      1. arise from previously normal skin.
      2. include fissures and excoriations.
      3. include lichenification and scars.
      4. evolve from consecutive changes in lesions.
      5. would include hives from an allergic reaction, for example.
   a) 1 and 5 are correct.
   b) 2 and 4 are correct.
   c) 1, 3 and 5 are correct.
   d) 2, 3 and 4 are correct.
   e) 1, 2 and 3 are correct.

20. Mr. Daniels, age 15, comes to the clinic complaining of itching facial lesions which
   developed during a camping trip. Your examination reveals three slightly irregular
   wheals, 0.05 to 1 cm in diameter, clustered on the left temporal area of the face. You
   would suspect
   a) poison oak.
   b) acne lesions.
   c) a systemic allergic reaction.
   d) insect bites.

Number 3
The Integument

RATIONALE

The purpose of this self-instructional unit is to help you learn inspection and palpation of the integument. The focus of this unit is on systematically identifying the normal characteristics of the skin, hair and nails and recognizing signs and symptoms which are considered abnormal. At the end of the unit you will be able to perform an examination of the integument, describe your findings and differentiate between normal and abnormal findings.

GLOSSARY OF TERMS

Review the following terms before and after completing this unit. You should be able to define or describe them readily.

Alopecia ____

Bulla ____

Crust ____

Erosion ____

Excoriation ____

Fissure ____

Furuncle ____

Keloid ____

Lichenification ____

Lipoma ____

Maceration ____

Macule ____

Nevus ____

Nodule ____

Papule ____

Plaque ____

Pruritus ____

Purpura ____

Pustule ____

Scale ____

Telangiectasia
   (cherry angioma, spider angioma) _______________________________________

Vesicle ____

Wheal ____

COGNITIVE OBJECTIVES

At the end of this unit you will demonstrate knowledge of inspection and palpation of the integument by your ability to:

1. List three functions of the integument.

2. Identify on a drawing the following structures of the skin: epidermis, dermis, subcutaneous tissue, sweat gland, sebaceous gland, hair follicle.

3. Differentiate between sebaceous, eccrine and apocrine glands.

4. Describe the effects of pigments, hemoglobin, bilirubin and vascular changes on skin coloration and describe purpuric and vascular lesions.

5. Define and give examples of different types of lesions.
   a. Primary: macule, papule, plaque, nodule, tumor, wheal, vesicle, bulla, pustule.
   b. Secondary: erosion, ulcer, fissure, crust, scale, lichenification, atrophy, excoriation, scar.

6. Explain the terms used in describing anatomical distribution of lesions — localized, generalized, contact, symmetrical — and give one common example of each.

7. Describe grouping configurations: linear, annular, clustered.

8. List causes of changes in skin moisture, temperature, texture, mobility and turgor.

9. Describe the normal appearance of nails and the significance of abnormal findings: color, shape, grooves, ridges, splinter hemorrhages and changes in the angle between the nail and finger.

10. Describe normal findings for assessing the hair: distribution and quantity over the scalp, pubic area and other areas of the body; texture and luster.

LEARNING ACTIVITIES

The Learning Activities contain information necessary for meeting the Cognitive Objectives. Select one and proceed to work with it until you have mastered the material. Use the Cognitive Objectives as a study guide. A Self-Test is provided so that you can check how much you know. If you have difficulty with the Self-Test, please review the material in this unit before proceeding to the Clinical Objectives.

Reading Activities

a) Bates: *A Guide to Physical Examination*, "The Skin." This chapter covers anatomy and physiology of the integument and examination techniques and contains useful tables of normal and abnormal findings for skin color, lesions and nail changes. You will need to supplement this activity by reading about assessment of hair characteristics.

b) DeGowin and DeGowin: *Bedside Diagnostic Examination*, "The Skin." This chapter presents detailed information on anatomy and physiology, examination techniques, morphology of lesions, hair characteristics and skin turgor. Emphasis is on abnormal findings.

c) Delp and Manning: *Major's Physical Diagnosis*, "Dermatology." Excellent photographs and descriptions of skin lesions are presented. The examination procedure is very well done. You will have to supplement your reading to meet the objectives.

d) Gillies and Alyn: *Patient Assessment and Management by the Nurse Practitioner.* Information about examination of the skin, hair and nails is integrated throughout the text.

e) Judge and Zuidema: *Methods of Clinical Examination: A Physiologic Approach*, "The Skin." This overview of assessment of the skin places emphasis on technique and normal findings. Cardinal symptoms and lesions are well described. You will need to supplement your reading to meet the objectives.

f) Prior and Silberstein: *Physical Diagnosis*, "Skin." This chapter contains information about anatomy and physiological functions of the integument including glands. Primary and secondary lesions are described in detail, as is skin coloration. Factors influencing skin moisture, texture, turgor and mobility and characteristics of hair are well presented. Supplement your reading to obtain details about distribution and configuration of lesions, purpuric and vascular lesions and nail characteristics.

g) Sana and Judge: *Physical Appraisal Methods in Nursing Practice*, "General Appearance and Skin Behavior." The section of this chapter which deals with skin discusses the anatomy and physiology of the skin, interviewing and physical appraisal guidelines, and the dermal appendages. You will need to supplement your reading with additional information about the nails, their characteristics, grouping and distribution of skin lesions and features of vascular lesions.

h) Sherman and Fields: *Guide to Patient Evaluation*, "The Integumentary System and Masses." This reading presents pertinent anatomy and physiology and then systematically describes techniques of examination. Tables of normal and abnormal findings are especially helpful. An example of the S.O.A.P. method of recording is also included.

Audiovisual Activities

(a) Blue-Hill Educational Systems, Inc.: "Integument," a 60-minute video tape program. This lecture encompasses anatomy and physiology of the integument as well as demonstrating inspection and palpation. There is detailed discussion of normal and abnormal findings for skin color, primary and secondary lesions, and hair and nail characteristics.

Supplemental Activity

The following material is suggested to supplement or strengthen your learning.

a) G. M. Levene and C. D. Calnan: *Color Atlas of Dermatology*. Chicago, Year Book Medical Publishers, Inc., 1974.

SELF-TEST

This Self-Test is for you. Use it to check how well you have learned the material presented in the unit. The answers follow the test.

1. Functions of the skin include
      1. protection.
      2. excretion.
      3. a sensory organ.
      4. temperature regulation.
   a) 1 only is correct.
   b) 4 only is correct.
   c) 1, 2 and 3 are correct.
   d) 2 and 4 are correct.
   e) all of the above are correct.

Identify the following structures of the skin, using the letters on the drawing:

2. _______ Arrector pili muscle

3. _______ Sweat gland

4. _______ Sebaceous gland

5. _______ Hair follicle

6. Skin pigments are formed in the _____________ layer of the skin.
   a) dermal
   b) epidermal
   c) subcutaneous
   d) vascular

7. Glands which help to control body temperature are called _____________ glands.
   a) apocrine
   b) sebaceous
   c) eccrine

8. Increased amounts of reduced hemoglobin circulating in the blood usually give light

   skin a _____________ appearance.
   a) flushed
   b) bluish
   c) yellowish
   d) very pale

9. An example of a lesion caused by blood escaping from a vessel would be
   a) a spider angioma.
   b) an erosion.
   c) a bulla.
   d) a petechia.

10. Primary lesions
    1. arise from previously normal skin.
    2. may be the initial manifestation of a disease.
    3. include such types as crusts and scales.
    4. include such types as macules and papules.
    5. would include the acne lesion.
    a) 1, 3 and 5 are correct.
    b) 1 only is correct.
    c) 3 only is correct.
    d) 1, 2, 4 and 5 are correct.
    e) all of the above are correct.

11. An area of thickened, rough skin with increased visibility of normal markings is called
    a) keloid.
    b) excoriation.
    c) atrophy.
    d) lichenification.
    e) scale.

12. The distribution pattern of lesions resulting from brushing your leg against poison oak leaves would be described as
    1. generalized.
    2. symmetrical.
    3. contact.
    4. localized.
    a) 3 and 4 are correct.
    b) 3 only is correct.
    c) 4 only is correct.
    d) 1 only is correct.
    e) 1 and 2 are correct.

13. The configuration for individual lesions arranged in circles or arcs, as occurs with urticaria, is called
    a) linear.
    b) clustered.
    c) annular.

14. Decreased skin turgor and/or mobility occurs in
    1. dehydration.
    2. rapid weight loss.
    3. fever.
    4. aged persons.
    5. edema.
    a) 1 only is correct.
    b) 2, 3 and 4 are correct.
    c) 1 and 4 are correct.
    d) 3 and 5 are correct.
    e) all of the above are correct.

Match each of the abnormal nail characteristics in items 15 through 18 with the most commonly associated pathological condition.

15. _______ Clubbing

16. _______ Spoon-shaped nails

17. _______ Splinter hemorrhages

18. _______ Beau's lines

a) Iron deficiency anemia
b) Subacute bacterial endocarditis
c) Acute, severe illness
d) Calcium deficiency
e) Chronic hypoxia

19. Conditions in which alopecia can occur include
    1. aging.
    2. hyperthyroidism.
    3. fever.
    4. heavy metal poisoning.
  a) 1 and 3 are correct.
  b) 2 and 4 are correct.
  c) 1, 3 and 4 are correct.
  d) all of the above are correct.

SELF-TEST KEY

1. (e) The skin and its secretions act as a barrier to chemical, thermal, mechanical and microbial injury. Glands and pores in the skin allow excretion of fluid and waste products. Numerous nerve endings provide receptors for sensory stimulation. The skin acts to dissipate internal heat and to insulate against external temperatures.

2. (c) Contraction of this muscle causes the hair to stand up.

3. (b) Coiled tubular gland which secretes perspiration.

4. (e) These specialized cells in the dermal lining of the hair follicle secrete oil.

5. (d) An invagination of skin layers; contains the hair shaft.

6. (b) Keratin and melanin are formed in the inner cellular layer of the epidermis. The dermis contains blood vessels, connective tissue and sebaceous glands. The subcutaneous layer contains hair follicles, sweat glands and fat.

7. (c) Evaporation of sweat from the eccrine glands helps to control body temperature. Sebaceous glands produce a fatty substance for lubrication and protection of hair and skin. Apocrine glands are modified sweat glands which respond to emotional, not thermal, stimuli.

8. (b) A large amount of reduced (unoxygenated) hemoglobin in the blood gives the skin a bluish appearance (cyanosis). Flushing or redness would be due to an increased visibility of oxygenated hemoglobin associated with dilatation of blood vessels in the skin or decreased tissue oxygen utilization. Jaundice results from an increased level of bilirubin, as occurs in hepatic disease. A very pale complexion may be caused by hypopigmentation or decreased visibility of the normal oxyhemoglobin.

9. (d) Petechiae are tiny reddish purple hemorrhages often due to increased bleeding tendencies. A spider angioma is a small vascular lesion, but the blood is contained within the vessel; they most frequently occur in pregnancy and hepatic disease. An erosion refers to loss of the superficial epidermis, usually without bleeding. A bulla is a large blister.

10. (d) Primary lesions occur in response to an exciting factor and may be the first indication of a disease process; examples are the macule (petechia), papule (insect bite) and pustule (acne). Crusts and scales are secondary changes that evolve from primary lesions.

11. (d) Keloid refers to a hypertrophied scar. Excoriations are scratch marks (pruritus). Atrophy refers to conditions in which the skin is thin and lacks the normal furrows (arterial insufficiency). Scales are flakes of skin (psoriasis).

12. (a) Generalized refers to distribution over most of the body. Symmetrical lesions are found on both sides of the body (drug-induced rashes). Poison oak lesions are localized to specific areas of direct contact with the plant.

13. (c) Linear configuration, as is typified by contact dermatitis, refers to a line of lesions. Clustered lesions occur in a group.

14. (e) Decreased elasticity of the skin occurs with dehydration states (fever), with senile cutaneous atrophy, and when there is rapid loss of body tissue. When edema is present, the underlying fluid decreases skin mobility.

15. (e)

16. (a)

17. (b)

18. (c)

19. (c) Hair loss may occur as physiological balding or as the result of fever, heavy metal poisoning, or hypothyroidism.

CLINICAL COMPONENT

Having completed the cognitive portion of this unit you are now ready to proceed to the Clinical Objectives. The purpose of the Clinical Component is to assess the integument and detect the presence, location and extent of any dysfunction.

CLINICAL OBJECTIVES

At the end of this unit you will perform an assessment of the integument, correlating physical examination skills with physiological principles. You will be able to:

1. Demonstrate knowledge of signs and symptoms of dysfunction related to the skin, hair and nails by obtaining a pertinent health history from the client.

2. Demonstrate inspection and palpation of the skin by assessing
   a. color – pigmentation, abnormal skin hues.
   b. vascularity – bleeding, bruising, lesions, cyanosis, pallor, flush.
   c. characteristics of lesions – type, grouping, distribution.
   d. moisture – dryness, sweating, oil.
   e. temperature.
   f. texture – rough, smooth.
   g. mobility and turgor.

3. Demonstrate inspection and palpation of the nails by assessing
   a. color.
   b. shape.
   c. angle.
   d. lesions.
   e. mobility.

4. Demonstrate inspection and palpation of the hair by assessing
   a. texture and luster.
   b. absence or excess.
   c. distribution.

5. Utilize S.O.A.P. to systematically describe findings, assess normality and formulate a plan for further action.

INSTRUCTIONS

Utilize three of your peers or clients in the clinical area to practice inspection and palpation of the integument. Remove the Performance Guide cards for Unit 3 from Appendix II. These cards will enable you to practice the skills necessary to meet the Clinical Objectives and complete the Response Sheets. On each Response Sheet you will be expected to (1) ask questions which elicit possible symptoms, (2) systematically describe your findings, (3) localize any abnormalities which are present and (4) summarize your examination findings using the S.O.A.P. method of recording.

When you have mastered the Clinical Objectives and completed the Response Sheets, arrange to demonstrate your skills to your laboratory instructor or preceptor.

EQUIPMENT

Drape
Flexible metric ruler
Gloves

OPTIONAL ACTIVITY

a) Blue-Hill Educational Systems, Inc.: "Integument and Lymph Nodes," an 18-minute video tape cassette. Techniques for assessment of the integument are demonstrated.

RESPONSE SHEET—INTEGUMENT

Client ___________________________________

Date _________________ Age _______ Sex _______

Examiner _________________________________

I. Health History

II. Physical Examination

   A. Skin

      1. Color

      2. Vascularity

      3. Moisture

      4. Temperature

      5. Texture

      6. Mobility/turgor

      7. Lesions

   B. Nails

      1. Color

      2. Shape

      3. Angle

      4. Mobility

      5. Lesions

C. Hair

1. Texture/luster

2. Absence/excess

3. Distribution

4. Scalp

Summarize your findings, using the S.O.A.P. method.

S. (Client's observations, complaints, health history)

O. (Physical findings)
Diagram any abnormalities on these outline drawings.

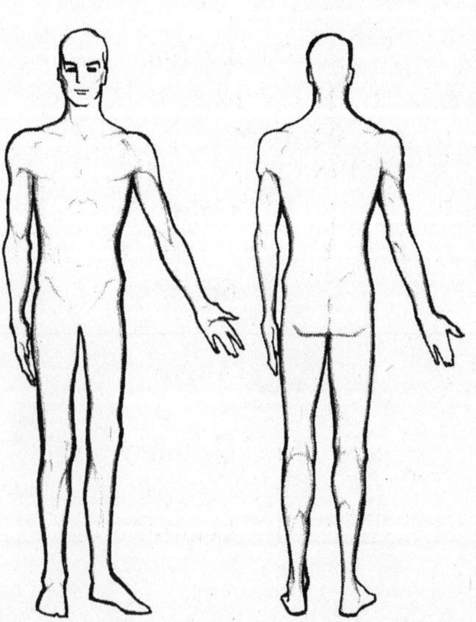

A. (Assessment of the problem, data, prognosis)

P. (Plans for further evaluation, care, teaching)

RESPONSE SHEET—INTEGUMENT

Client _______________________________

Date _________________ Age _______ Sex _______

Examiner _____________________________

I. Health History

II. Physical Examination

   A. Skin

      1. Color

      2. Vascularity

      3. Moisture

      4. Temperature

      5. Texture

      6. Mobility/turgor

      7. Lesions

   B. Nails

      1. Color

      2. Shape

      3. Angle

      4. Mobility

      5. Lesions

C. Hair

    1. Texture/luster

    2. Absence/excess

    3. Distribution

    4. Scalp

Summarize your findings, using the S.O.A.P. method.

S. **(Client's observations, complaints, health history)**

O. **(Physical findings)**
Diagram any abnormalities on these outline drawings.

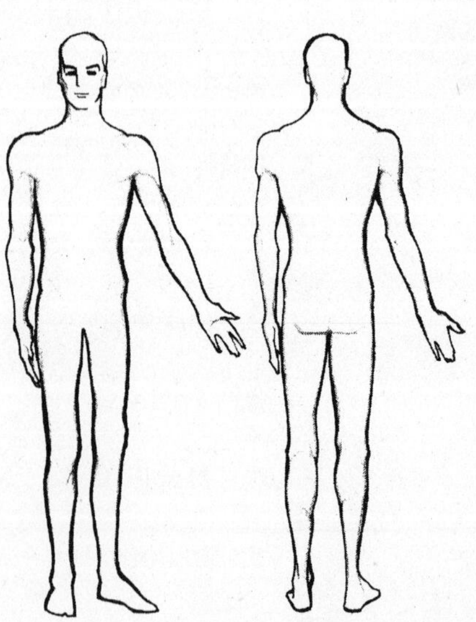

A. (Assessment of the problem, data, prognosis)

P. (Plans for further evaluation, care, teaching)

RESPONSE SHEET—INTEGUMENT

Client _______________________________

Date _______________ Age ______ Sex ______

Examiner _____________________________

I. Health History

II. Physical Examination

A. Skin

1. Color

2. Vascularity

3. Moisture

4. Temperature

5. Texture

6. Mobility/turgor

7. Lesions

B. Nails

1. Color

2. Shape

3. Angle

4. Mobility

5. Lesions

C. Hair

    1. Texture/luster

    2. Absence/excess

    3. Distribution

    4. Scalp

Summarize your findings, using the S.O.A.P. method.

S. (Client's observations, complaints, health history)

O. (Physical findings)
Diagram any abnormalities on these outline drawings.

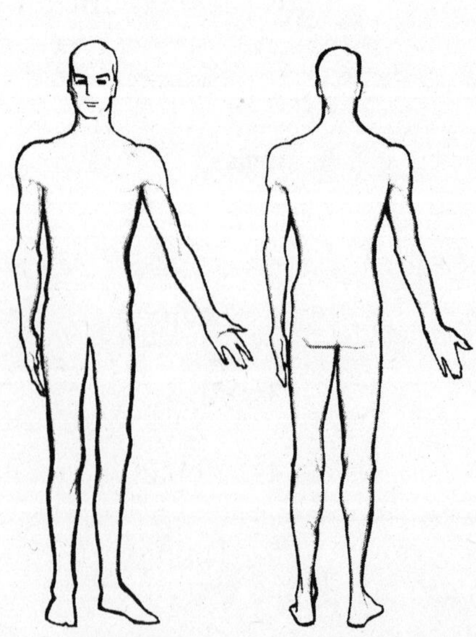

A. (Assessment of the problem, data, prognosis)

P. (Plans for further evaluation, care, teaching)

PRE-TEST

UNIT 4

Choose the *one* best answer.

1. Pulse pressure is
   a) the highest pressure palpated in the arteries.
   b) the lowest pressure palpated in the arteries.
   c) the difference between systolic and diastolic pressures.
   d) the average pressure palpated in the arteries.

2. A bounding pulse
   1. is associated with a wide pulse pressure.
   2. can be seen.
   3. has a fast upbeat and drop.
   4. is associated with shock.
   a) all of the above are correct.
   b) 1, 2, and 3 are correct.
   c) 2 and 3 are correct.
   d) 3 and 4 are correct.

3. Arterial insufficiency is characterized by
   1. loss of hair.
   2. atrophic skin.
   3. decreased or absent pulses.
   4. increased venous filling time.
   a) 1 and 2 are correct.
   b) 2, 3 and 4 are correct.
   c) all of the above are correct.
   d) 3 only is correct.

4. The jugular veins are used to evaluate
   a) increased left atrial pressures.
   b) venous pressure and pulsations.
   c) increased left ventricular pressures.
   d) none of the above.

5. Pulsus alterans is characterized by
   1. regular rhythm.
   2. decreased amplitude on inspiration.
   3. alternating large and small amplitude beats.
   4. coupling of two beats with the second beat.
   a) 1 and 2 are correct.
   b) 3 only is correct.
   c) 1 and 4 are correct.
   d) 1 and 3 are correct.

6. A narrowed pulse pressure, jugular venous distention, peripheral cyanosis and decreased mentation indicate the client has
   a) decreased cardiac pumping action.
   b) orthostatic hypotension.
   c) both a and b.
   d) neither a nor b.

7. Homans' sign is characterized by
   a) calf pain on sharp dorsiflexion of the foot with the knee slightly bent.
   b) pain when the calf is squeezed gently.
   c) calf pain on sharp plantar flexion of the foot.
   d) diminished or absent pulses.

8. A small blood pressure cuff or one that is applied too loosely will
   a) give a falsely high reading.
   b) give a falsely low reading.
   c) not affect the reading.

9. A decreased or narrowed pulse pressure may result from
   a) a narrowed aortic or pulmonary valve.
   b) decreased myocardial contractility.
   c) both of the above.

Locate the following arterial pulses on the accompanying diagram:

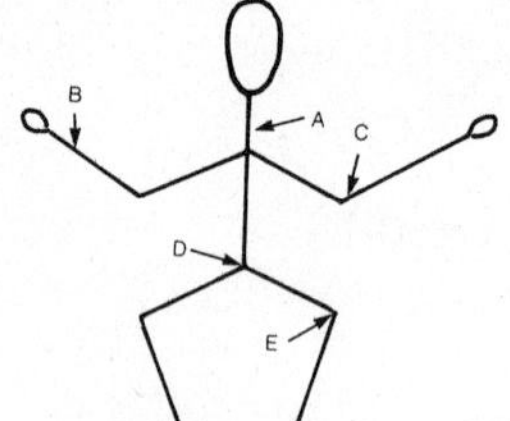

10. _________ Popliteal

11. _________ Brachial

12. Arterial pulses are evaluated for
    a) rate, rhythm and amplitude.
    b) amplitude and character.
    c) rate, rhythm, amplitude, contour and equality.
    d) rate, contour, amplitude and character.

13. "Auscultatory gap" refers to
    a) the 4th Korotkoff sound.
    b) the fact that sounds may disappear between the systolic and diastolic pressures and then reappear.
    c) a falsely high blood pressure reading.
    d) the disappearance of sound after the diastolic reading.

14. Jugular venous pressure is increased by
    a) right-sided heart failure.
    b) expiration.
    c) ascites.
    d) all of the above.

Mark (a) for True and (b) for False.

15. _______ A slow rising, slow falling carotid impulse is palpated in aortic stenosis.

16. _______ Sinus arrhythmia always represents a diseased myocardium.

17. _______ The systolic blood pressure in the lower extremities is usually about 10 mm Hg above that in the upper extremities.

18. _______ Venous neck pulsations can easily be occluded by light pressure.

19. _______ Endocrine disorders are the basis of essential hypertension.

20. _______ Diastole represents ventricular contraction.

Number 4

The Peripheral Vascular System

RATIONALE

This self-instructional unit is designed to help you learn inspection, palpation and auscultation of the peripheral arterial and venous circulation. The unit concentrates on evaluation of blood pressure and arterial and venous pulsations. At the end of the unit you will be able to systematically describe normal and abnormal findings as they relate to blood pressure and arterial and venous pulsations.

GLOSSARY OF TERMS

In order to complete this unit you should be familiar with the following terms:

Arrhythmia ____

Bradycardia ____

Bruit ____

Cyanosis ____

Diastole ____

Hepatojugular reflux (HJR) ____

Homans' sign ____

Hypertension ____

Korotkoff sounds ____

Orthostatic hypotension ____

Pulse pressure ____

Pulsus alternans ____

Pulsus paradoxus ____

Sinus arrhythmia ____

Systole____

Tachycardia____

Thrombophlebitis____

Varicose____

Venous hum____

COGNITIVE OBJECTIVES

At the end of this unit you will demonstrate knowledge of inspection and palpation of the peripheral cardiovascular system by your ability to:

1. Define and give an example of systolic pressure, diastolic pressure, pulse pressure and mean pressure.

2. List and define the five phases of the Korotkoff method for auscultating blood pressure.

3. Identify the normal range of systolic and diastolic pressures in the limbs.

4. Identify some of the abnormal conditions which cause
    a. an increased systolic pressure.
    b. an increased diastolic pressure.
    c. a widened pulse pressure.
    d. a narrowed pulse pressure.

5. Locate on a diagram the anatomical position of the carotid, brachial, radial, femoral, popliteal, dorsalis pedis and posterior tibial pulses.

6. Describe the normal rate, rhythm, amplitude and contour of the arterial pulse.

7. Describe the following abnormal pulses: bounding pulse, pulsus alternans, pulsus paradoxus and slow rising (small) pulse. List one causative factor for each.

8. Describe the normal findings of venous neck pulsations and pressure during inspection.

9. Identify the implications of jugular venous distention and abnormal venous pulsations.

10. List observations which indicate arterial insufficiency.

11. Identify signs of superficial and deep vein thrombosis.

LEARNING ACTIVITIES

The Learning Activities contain the information necessary for meeting the Cognitive Objectives. Select one and proceed to work with it until you have mastered the material. Use the Cognitive Objectives as a study guide. A Self-Test is provided so you can check how much you know. If you have difficulty with the Self-Test, please review the material in this unit before proceeding to the Clinical Objectives.

Reading Activities

a) Bates: *A Guide to Physical Examination*, "Pressures and Pulses: Arterial and Venous" and "The Peripheral Vascular System." These chapters provide an excellent description of jugular venous pressure and pulse. Measurement of blood pressure is well illustrated. Anatomy and physiology of arterial pressures and pulse are described clearly, but the student will need to do additional readings for definitions and abnormalities of blood pressure.

b) Delp and Manning: *Major's Physical Diagnosis*, "Blood Pressure and Pulse" and "Peripheral Vascular Disease." Methods of determining blood pressure, normal and abnormal values are clearly outlined. Characteristics of arterial pulse and irregularities are discussed in depth. These chapters have a strong disease orientation and assume a working knowledge of anatomy and physiology.

c) DeGowin and DeGowin: *Bedside Diagnostic Examination*, "The Blood Vessels." This chapter offers a comprehensive discussion of blood pressure and arterial pulses. Venous pulsations are well described and diagrammed; however, discussion of venous neck pressure measurement is unclear. Abnormalities of peripheral circulation are presented in great detail. Scan the material to identify information needed to meet the objectives.

d) Gillies and Alyn: *Patient Assessment and Management by the Nurse Practitioner*. The information for meeting the objectives is difficult to retrieve from this text. The discussion of pulse in Chapter 3 is related to the examination of the neck and the extremities. Blood pressure determination is discussed in Chapter 7. Additional readings are recommended.

e) Judge and Zuidema: *Methods of Clinical Examination: A Physiologic Approach*, "Circulatory System." Techniques for assessing blood pressure, arterial pulses, venous neck pulsations and pressures are clearly described in the chapters. Normal and abnormal findings are related to underlying physiological mechanisms.

f) Prior and Silberstein: *Physical Diagnosis*, "The Cardiovascular System." This chapter presents much of the information needed to meet the Cognitive Objectives. Additional reading for clarification may be necessary. The student will have to refer to Chapter 14 ("Extremities") for observations related to arterial and venous abnormalities.

g) Sana and Judge: *Physical Appraisal Methods in Nursing Practice*, "Physical Appraisal of Circulatory Function." Assessment of blood pressure is covered fully. Observations related to characteristics of arterial pulses are presented superficially; measurement of venous neck pressure is omitted. Common abnormalities are well described.

h) Sherman and Fields: *Guide to Patient Evaluation*. Evaluation of the peripheral cardiovascular system is not specifically presented in this text.

Audiovisual Activities

a) Blue-Hill Educational Systems, Inc.: "Cardiovascular System – Peripheral Circulation," Tape 12A. The lecture includes a discussion of blood pressure, inspection and palpation of arterial pulses and signs of arterial insufficiency, and it concludes with evaluation of neck veins and peripheral veins.

Supplemental Activity

Read the following material to strengthen your learning.

a) Frank and Alvarez-Mena: *Cardiovascular Physical Diagnosis*. This modified programmed instruction presents material on blood pressure, inspection and palpation of arterial and venous pulsations.

SELF-TEST

The Self-Test is for you. Use it to check how well you have learned the material in the unit. The answers are provided in the Self-Test Key which follows.

1. The pulse pressure
   a) measures the force of left ventricular contraction.
   b) is the average pressure in the arterial system.
   c) is the difference between the diastolic and systolic pressures.
   d) measures peripheral vascular resistance.

2. List the five phases of the Korotkoff method for auscultating blood pressure

   a) _______________________   d) _______________________

   b) _______________________   e) _______________________

   c) _______________________

3. The palpated systolic pressure
   a) is usually lower than the auscultated systolic pressure.
   b) should always be obtained before the systolic pressure is auscultated.
   c) both of the above are correct.
   d) neither of the above is correct.

Mark items 4 through 10 (a) for True or (b) for False.

4. _______ Blood pressure is normally somewhat higher in the popliteal artery than in the brachial artery.

5. _______ Blood pressure normally drops for a moment when a patient stands from a sitting or supine position.

6. _______ The pulse pressure is narrowed in hyperthyroidism and emotional states.

7. _______ An elevated diastolic pressure results in greater stress to the cardiovascular system than isolated systolic hypertension.

8. _______ Pulsus paradoxus is an important sign of cardiac tamponade or constrictive pericarditis.

9. _______ Pulsus bigeminus has a regular rhythm but the pulse force alternates between strong and weak beats.

10. _______ Jugular veins normally fill above the clavicle when the client is at a 45° angle.

11. Arterial insufficiency is characterized by
    1. hair loss.
    2. shiny atrophic skin.
    3. long venous filling time.
    4. decreased or absent pulses.
  a) 4 only is correct.
  b) 1, 2 and 4 are correct.
  c) 2, 3 and 4 are correct.
  d) all of the above are correct.

12. Homans' sign is used to elicit
  a) venous pulsations.
  b) deep thrombophlebitis.
  c) varicosities.
  d) all of the above.

SELF-TEST KEY

1. (c) The pulse pressure is defined as the difference in mm Hg between the systolic and diastolic pressures. The systolic pressure measures the force of left ventricular contraction; the diastolic pressure is a measure of peripheral vascular resistance; and the mean pressure is the average pressure in the arterial system.

2. The five phases of the Korotkoff sounds are (a) phase one – onset of sound, (b) phase two – no sound (auscultatory gap), (c) phase three – distinct sound, (d) phase four – muffled sound and (e) phase five – disappearance of sound.

3. (c) The palpated systolic pressure is usually 10 to 15 mm Hg lower than the auscultated systolic pressure. Occasionally the palpated pressure is higher, and therefore, the systolic pressure should be palpated before auscultation.

4. (a) True. The systolic blood pressure is normally 10 mm Hg higher in the lower extremities than in the upper extremities.

5. (a) True. When a client assumes an erect position the systolic pressure may drop by 10 to 15 mg Hg, and in about half the cases the diastolic pressure will rise slightly.

6. (b) False. A narrowed pulse pressure is seen with a decrease in stroke volume as in tachycardia or congestive heart failure. Hyperthyroidism and emotional states usually increase the stroke volume and therefore widen the pulse pressure.

7. (a) True. The diastolic pressure is the least pressure exerted by the blood against the wall of the vessel. Therefore, an increase in the diastolic pressure results in an overall increase of pressures on the vessel walls.

8. (a) True. Pulsus paradoxus is found with pericardial effusions and with constrictive pericarditis. The systolic blood pressure falls with inspiration. Venous return is increased normally with inspiration. However, the heart is constricted, and diastolic filling is decreased with a concomitant fall in systolic blood pressure. In pulsus paradoxus, the systolic pressure usually falls by 10 mm Hg or more with inspiration.

9. (b) False. Pulsus alternans has a regular rhythm, but the force of the pulse alternates between strong and weak beats. Pulsus bigeminus is a coupling of two beats separated by a pause.

10. (b) False. At a 45° angle the jugular vein is normally flat at the level of the clavicle. This is due to the effect of gravity.

11. (d) Arterial insufficiency may be due to degenerative or inflammatory processes in the vessel wall. It is characterized by diminished or absent pulses; loss of hair; atrophy of muscles and soft tissues; shiny, taut, scaly skin; a feeling of coolness; and an increased venous filling time.

12. (b) Deep venous thrombosis may be suspected when the client complains of calf pain or dorsiflexion of the foot with the knee slightly flexed (Homans' sign).

CLINICAL COMPONENT

Having completed the cognitive portion of this unit you are now ready to proceed to the Clinical Objectives. The purpose of the Clinical Component is to assess the peripheral cardiovascular system for normal configuration and detect the presence, location and extent of any dysfunction.

CLINICAL OBJECTIVES

At the end of this unit you will be able to perform assessment of the peripheral cardiovascular system, correlating physical examination skills with physiological principles. You will be able to:

1. Demonstrate knowledge of signs and symptoms of dysfunction related to the peripheral cardiovascular system by obtaining a pertinent health history from the client.

2. Demonstrate palpation and auscultation of blood pressure and accurately record findings.

3. Demonstrate inspection and palpation of the carotid artery by recording rate, rhythm, amplitude, symmetry and contour.

4. Demonstrate inspection and palpation of the internal jugular vein by recording
    a. amplitude and contour.
    b. distention – direction of blood flow, hepatojugular reflux.

5. Demonstrate palpation of peripheral arterial pulses (brachial, radial, femoral, popliteal, dorsalis pedis and posterior tibial) by
    a. recording amplitude and symmetry.
    b. identifying signs of arterial insufficiency.

6. Demonstrate inspection and palpation of peripheral veins by recording signs of venous insufficiency.

7. Utilize S.O.A.P. to systematically describe findings, make an assessment regarding normality and formulate a plan of action.

INSTRUCTIONS

Utilizing three of your peers or clients in the clinical area, practice inspection, palpation and auscultation of the peripheral cardiovascular system. Remove the Performance Guide cards for Unit 4 from Appendix II. These cards will enable you to practice the skills necessary to meet the Clinical Objectives and complete the Response Sheets. On each Response Sheet you will be expected to (1) ask questions which elicit possible symptoms, (2) systematically describe your findings, (3) localize any abnormalities that are present and (4) summarize your examination findings using the S.O.A.P. method of recording.

When you have mastered the Clinical Objectives and completed the Response Sheets, arrange to demonstrate your skills to your laboratory instructor or preceptor.

EQUIPMENT

Blood pressure cuff — arm and thigh
Examining table, bed or pillows to elevate head of bed to 45° angle
Gooseneck lamp or flashlight to provide tangential lighting
Stethoscope with diaphragm and bell
Tape measure

ACTIVITIES

The following Bates' films demonstrate the techniques of peripheral cardiovascular assessment.

a) "Pressures and Pulses: Arterial and Venous" demonstrates examination of blood pressure and neck vessels.

b) "The Peripheral Vascular System" presents the evaluation of peripheral pulses and adequacy of blood flow to the extremities.

RESPONSE SHEET—THE PERIPHERAL VASCULAR SYSTEM

Client _______________________________________

Date _____________________ Age _______ Sex _______

Examiner _______________________________________

I. Health History

II. Physical Examination (Describe findings, diagram abnormalities)

A. Blood Pressure (repeat if elevated)

	sitting	standing	lying	(thigh)
L				
R				

B. Neck Vessels

1. Carotid artery

   a. Inspection:

   b. Palpation:

2. Internal jugular vein

   a. Inspection:

   b. Palpation:

C. Peripheral Vessels

1. Arteries

   a. Inspection:

   b. Palpation: Rate _________ Rhythm _________

	brachial	radial	femoral	popliteal	D. pedis	P. tibialis
L						
R						

   0 = absent;   1+ = weak;   2+ = normal;   3+ = strong;   4+ = bounding

2. Veins

   a. Inspection:

   b. Palpation:

Summarize your findings using the S.O.A.P. method.

S.   (Client's observations, complaints, health history)

O.   (Physical findings)
Diagram the client's pulses on the accompanying drawing.

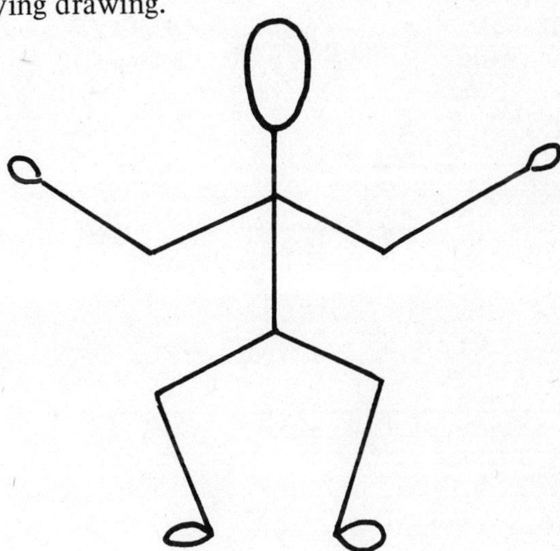

A.   (Assessment of the problem, data, prognosis)

P.   (Plans for further evaluation, care, teaching)

Client _______________________________

Date _________________ Age ________ Sex ________

Examiner _______________________________

I. Health History

II. Physical Examination (Describe findings, diagram abnormalities)

A. Blood Pressure (repeat if elevated)

	sitting	standing	lying	(thigh)
L				
R				

B. Neck Vessels

1. Carotid artery

   a. Inspection:

   b. Palpation:

2. Internal jugular vein

   a. Inspection:

   b. Palpation:

C. Peripheral Vessels

1. Arteries

    a. Inspection:

    b. Palpation: Rate _________ Rhythm _________

	brachial	radial	femoral	popliteal	D. pedis	P. tibialis
L						
R						

0 = absent; 1+ = weak; 2+ = normal; 3+ = strong; 4+ = bounding

2. Veins

    a. Inspection:

    b. Palpation:

Summarize your findings using the S.O.A.P. method.

S. **(Client's observations, complaints, health history)**

O. **(Physical findings)**
Diagram the client's pulses on the accompanying drawing.

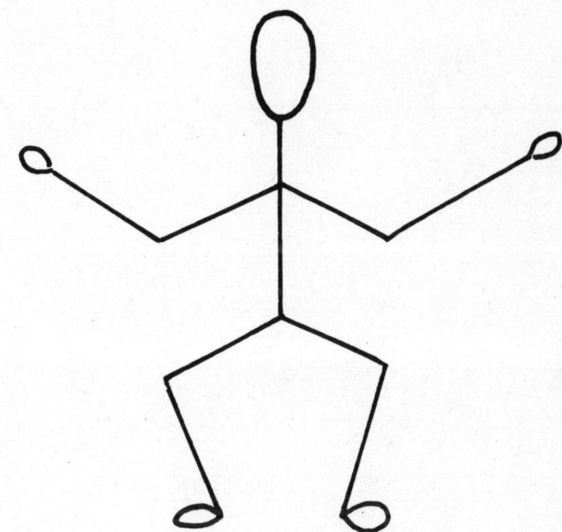

A. **(Assessment of the problem, data, prognosis)**

P. **(Plans for further evaluation, care, teaching)**

Client _______________________________

Date _____________________ Age _______ Sex _______

Examiner _______________________________

I. Health History

II. Physical Examination (Describe findings, diagram abnormalities)

A. Blood Pressure (repeat if elevated)

	sitting	standing	lying	(thigh)
L				
R				

B. Neck Vessels

1. Carotid artery

   a. Inspection:

   b. Palpation:

2. Internal jugular vein

   a. Inspection:

   b. Palpation:

C. Peripheral Vessels

1. Arteries

   a. Inspection:

   b. Palpation: Rate _________ Rhythm _________

	brachial	radial	femoral	popliteal	D. pedis	P. tibialis
L						
R						

   0 = absent; 1+ = weak; 2+ = normal; 3+ = strong; 4+ = bounding

2. Veins

   a. Inspection:

   b. Palpation:

Summarize your findings using the S.O.A.P. method.

S. (Client's observations, complaints, health history)

O. (Physical findings)
Diagram the client's pulses on the accompanying drawing.

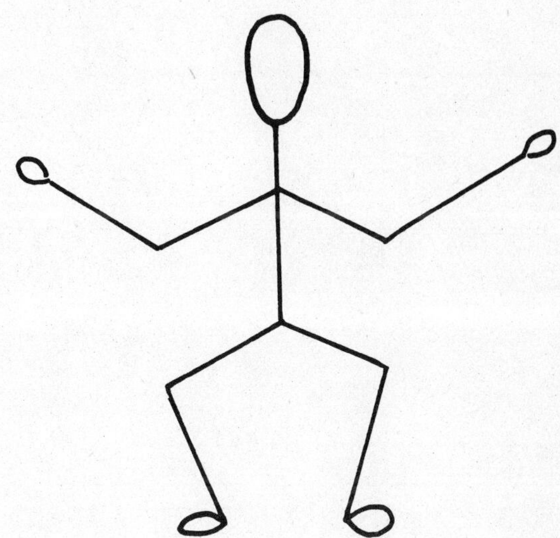

A. (Assessment of the problem, data, prognosis)

P. (Plans for further evaluation, care, teaching)

UNIT 5

Match the following columns – one answer for items 1 through 3.

1. _______ Kyphosis   a) Lateral spinal curve
       b) Shortening of the sternocleidomastoid muscle

2. _______ Lordosis   c) Exaggerated lumbar spinal curve
       d) Exaggerated thoracic spinal curve

3. _______ Scoliosis

4. Five *major* factors used to assess gait are
    1. stance.
    2. step length.
    3. tendency to fall or stagger.
    4. arm swing.
    5. weight and height.
    6. need to watch feet.
    7. age.
   a) 1, 2, 3, 4 and 5 are correct.
   b) 2, 3, 5, 6 and 7 are correct.
   c) 1, 2, 3, 4 and 6 are correct.

5. A propulsive gait is common in
   a) cerebral palsy.
   b) tabes dorsalis.
   c) Parkinson's disease

6. An ataxic gait is characterized by
   a) cerebral disease.
   b) staggering or reeling.
   c) spasticity.
   d) paralysis of the adductor thigh muscles.

7. Painless nodules commonly found on the tendon sheaths of the wrists are
   a) ganglia.
   b) tophi.
   c) rheumatoid nodules.

Mark (a) for True or (b) for False in items 8 through 13.

8. _______ Ligament tears result in decreased passive range of motion.

9. _______ Flaccid paralysis results in a scissors gait.

10. _______ Parkinson's disease is characterized by wide stance, eyes on the ground, feet raised high and slapped on the ground.

11. _______ Crepitation refers to vibrations heard or felt over a joint.

12. _______ Ankylosis is a fracture of the ankle bones.

13. _______ Abduction is movement toward the body.

14. A circumductive gait is characteristic of
    a) hemiplegia.
    b) cerebral palsy.
    c) Parkinson's disease.
    d) cerebellar disease.

15. Talipes equinovarus is
    a) flat feet.
    b) high arches.
    c) angulation of the foot toward the midline of the body.
    d) club foot.
    e) webbed toes.

16. While examining a client's knees, you notice that one of them appears to be slightly swollen. This could be the result of
    1. bony enlargement.
    2. increased fluid in the bursa.
    3. a thickened synovial membrane.
    a) 2 only is correct.
    b) 2 and 3 are correct.
    c) 1 and 3 are correct.
    d) 1 and 2 are correct.
    e) all of the above are correct.

17. The dorsum of the foot is the _______ side.
    a) bottom
    b) medial
    c) top
    d) lateral

18. Having a client bend forward and touch the toes is done
    1. to check spinal ROM.
    2. with the examiner standing in front of the client.
    3. to make spinal deformities more obvious to detection.
    4. with the examiner behind the client.
    5. to check balance.
    a) 1, 2 and 3 are correct.
    b) 1, 3 and 4 are correct.
    c) 1 and 2 are correct.
    d) 3, 4 and 5 are correct.
    e) all of the above are correct.

19. A client with Dupuytren's contracture will be unable to
    a) flex the fourth and fifth fingers.
    b) abduct the thumb.
    c) make a fist.

d) extend the fourth and fifth fingers.
e) point with the first finger.

20. One way to assess rotation of the hip is to flex the client's knee, place the foot on the opposite patella and move the knee laterally and medially.
a) True
b) False

Number 5

The Musculoskeletal System

RATIONALE

The purpose of this self-instructional unit is to help you learn inspection and palpation of the musculoskeletal system. Primary emphasis is on observation of gait; symmetry of bones, joints and muscles; and range of motion. After completing the unit you will be able to systematically assess and describe a client's gait, body symmetry and range of motion and to make judgments regarding normality.

GLOSSARY OF TERMS

Review the following terms before and after completing this unit. You should be able to define or describe them readily.

Abduction ____

Adduction ____

Ankylosing spondylitis ____

Ankylosis ____

Ataxia ____

Bursa ____

Circumduction ____

Crepitation ____

Dorsal ____

Dupuytren's contracture ____

Eversion ____

Gait ____

Ganglion ____

Hallux valgus ____

Kyphosis ____

Lordosis ____

Nodule ____

Olecranon process ____

Patella ____

Pes planus ____

Plantar ____

Range of motion (ROM) ____

Rheumatoid ____

Sciatica ____

Scoliosis ____

Steppage ____

Talipes equinovarus ____

Torticollis ____

COGNITIVE OBJECTIVES

At the end of this unit you will demonstrate knowledge of inspection and palpation of the musculoskeletal system by your ability to:

1. Describe the following abnormalities and compare them with normal spinal curvature: lordosis, kyphosis, scoliosis, ankylosing spondylitis.

2. Describe factors used to assess gait: stance, step size, balance, arm swing, need to watch feet.

3. Discuss the etiology and characteristics of the following abnormal gaits: wide steppage (slapping), ataxic, scissors, circumducted (dragging), and Parkinsonian.

4. Discuss symptoms, causative factors and clinical implications of asymmetry of bones, joints and muscles.

5. Describe procedures for determining active and passive range of motion for each body part and identify factors which increase or decrease normal ROM.

6. Explain crepitation and describe how it is detected.

LEARNING ACTIVITIES

The Learning Activities contain the information necessary for meeting the Cognitive Objectives. Select one and proceed to work with it until you have mastered the material. Use the Cognitive Objectives as a study guide. A Self-Test is provided so that you can check how much you know. If you have difficulty with the Self-Test please review the material in this unit before proceeding to the Clinical Objectives.

Reading Activities

a) Bates: *A Guide to Physical Examination*, pp. 226–248, provides a discussion of the anatomy and physiology and techniques of examination of the musculoskeletal system (omit bulge sign and ballottement on p. 245). See pp. 251–262 for common abnormalities. Continue reading on the top of p. 276 and on pp. 299–300 for a discussion of gaits. The author proceeds to explain and illustrates each gait.

b) DeGowin and DeGowin: *Bedside Diagnostic Examination*, "The Spine and Extremities," presents very detailed examinations and findings for the bones and joints. Use the study guide to glean the information necessary to meet the Cognitive Objectives. Abnormal gaits are discussed in the chapter on neurological assessment.

c) Delp and Manning: *Major's Physical Diagnosis*, Chapter 12, "Examination of the Back and Extremities." This chapter discusses in detail gait and stance, and normal and abnormal findings of bones, joints and muscles; it also provides diagrams for testing range of motion. Numerous photographs aid understanding.

d) Gillies and Alyn: *Patient Assessment and Management by the Nurse Practitioner*. Information about the musculoskeletal system is integrated throughout the text, specifically in Chapter 3, on neurological examination, the back and the extremities.

e) Judge and Zuidema: *Methods of Clinical Examination: A Physiologic Approach*, "The Musculoskeletal System," assumes familiarity with anatomy and physiology. Normal and abnormal findings are integrated into descriptions of examination procedures. This text includes a helpful glossary of relevant terminology, but information about gaits must be obtained from another source.

f) Prior and Silberstein: *Physical Diagnosis*, Chapter 16, "Musculoskeletal System." General examination including an overview of gaits, deformities, measurement and joint evaluation and range of motion is followed by discussion of specific parts. Supplement your learning with additional reading about Parkinson's, wide-steppage, and circumducted gaits.

g) Sana and Judge: *Physical Appraisal Methods in Nursing Practice*, Chapter 13, "Detection of Aberrations in Neuromuscular Functioning," presents an overview of assessment of joint function. Supplement in all areas to meet the Cognitive Objectives.

h) Sherman and Fields: *Guide to Patient Evaluation*, "The Extremities and the Back," presents an overview of the musculoskeletal examination and will need supplementation in all areas. Some abnormalities of gait are presented clearly in table form.

Audiovisual Activities

a) Blue-Hill Educational Systems, Inc.: "Musculoskeletal System" (video tape 16) begins with an in-depth presentation of gait and abnormalities of gait. The lecturer then considers symmetry and asymmetry of the spine, extremities and muscles.

Supplemental Activities

The following activities are suggested to supplement or strengthen your learning.

a) "Scoliosis," Clinical Symposium. Reprints available from CIBA Pharmaceutical Co.

b) "Rheumatoid Arthritis," Clinical Symposium. Reprints available from CIBA Pharmaceutical Co.

SELF-TEST

This Self-Test is for you. Use it to check how well you have learned the material presented in the unit. The answers follow the test.

1. Draw and label the normal spinal curvatures.

2. Abnormal lateral curving of the spine is called
    a) lordosis.
    b) scoliosis.
    c) torticollis.
    d) kyphosis.
    e) ankylosis.

3. List five major factors used to assess gait.

    a) ________________________   d) ________________________

    b) ________________________   e) ________________________

    c) ________________________

4. Define steppage.

5. An ataxic gait due to cerebellar disease is characterized by
    a) spasticity.
    b) narrow stance.
    c) staggering or reeling.
    d) propulsive movements.

6. A dragging or circumductive gait is common in
    a) hemiplegia.
    b) cerebral palsy.

    c) Parkinson's disease.
    d) cerebellar disease.

7. Joint swelling or deformity may be caused by
    a) thickened synovial membrane.
    b) fluid in the joint capsule.
    c) bony enlargement.
    d) all of the above.

8. Dorsiflexion and plantar flexion are motions associated with the
    a) patella.
    b) foot.
    c) femur.
    d) shoulder.

9. The abnormal abduction of the big toe in relation to the first metatarsal is known as
    a) hammer toe.
    b) talipes equinovarus.
    c) pes planus.
    d) hallux valgus.

SELF-TEST KEY

1.

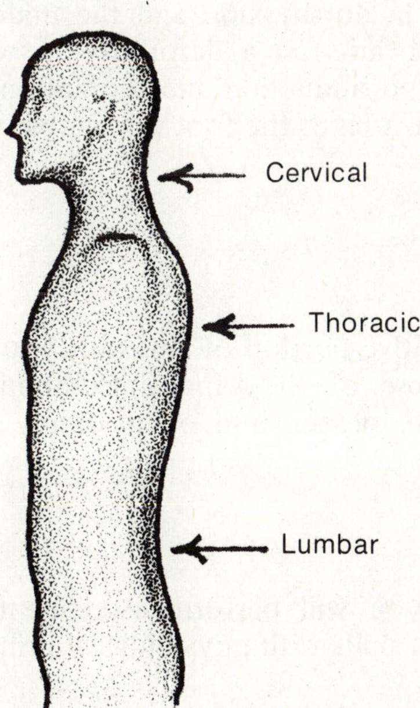

2. (b) Scoliosis is an abnormal lateral spinal curvature. With lordosis the normal anterior lumbar curve is exaggerated (sway back). Torticollis is a shortening of the neck muscles on one side. Kyphosis is an exaggeration of the normal posterior thoracic convexity. Ankylosis refers to an abnormal fusion of a joint.

3. Stance, length of step, balance, rhythmic arm swing, starting and stopping.

4. Steppage is the way in which the client lifts each foot, transfers weight and then places the foot back on the ground.

5. (c) Cerebellar ataxia results in an unsteady, wide-based gait most characterized by a staggering or reeling nature. With spasticity, as in bilateral spastic paresis of the legs, the thighs are adducted and the knees rub against each other in a scissors-like fashion. Propulsive movements are characteristic with the parkinsonian gait (see answer to 6) in which the body is propelled forward.

6. (a) With paralysis of one side, the affected leg is pulled out, around and forward in a circle or arc. Cerebral palsy is commonly associated with slow, writhing involuntary movements of the body. In Parkinson's disease, the gait abnormality consists of a forward projected torso, decreased arm swing and short, shuffling steps. Cerebellar disease is characterized by staggering or reeling (see answer to 5).

7. (d) An enlarged joint due to swelling or deformity can occur with thickening of the synovial membrane (as in rheumatoid arthritis), fluid in the synovial cavity (trauma, inflammation) or bony enlargement (osteoarthritis).

8. (b) Dorsiflexion and plantar flexion are terms used to describe the upward and downward flexions of the foot. The top of the foot is the dorsal surface, the bottom is the plantar surface. The patella or knee is primarily flexed and extended. The femur (long bone of the thigh) is not bendable. The shoulder represents a ball-and-socket joint capable of movement in many directions.

9. (d) Hammer toe often accompanies hallux valgus and is the condition in which the proximal joint is fixed in dorsiflexion and the middle joint fixed in plantar flexion. Clubfoot (talipes equinovarus) is a deformity in which there is varus of the heel, equinus of the ankle, and adduction and supination of the forefoot. Pes planus (flat foot) is present when the arch of the foot is lowered.

CLINICAL COMPONENT

Having completed the cognitive portion of this unit you are now ready to proceed to the Clinical Objectives. The purpose of the Clinical Component is to assess musculoskeletal function and detect the presence, location and extent of any dysfunction.

CLINICAL OBJECTIVES

At the end of this unit you will perform assessment of the musculoskeletal system correlating physical examination skills with physiological principles. You will be able to:

1. Demonstrate knowledge of signs and symptoms of dysfunction related to the musculoskeletal system by obtaining a pertinent health history from the client.

2. Demonstrate inspection of the musculoskeletal system by assessing
   a. posture and gait.
   b. ability of the client to carry out the activities of daily living.
   c. bones, joints and muscles for symmetry, color, swelling, nodules, deformities and atrophy.

3. Demonstrate palpation by assessing
   a. the head, spine and extremities for deviation from or limitation in normal range of motion.

    b. crepitation on movement of joints.
    c. tenderness or deformity of joints.
    d. muscle size.
    e. subcutaneous nodules.

4. Utilize S.O.A.P. to systematically describe findings, make an assessment of musculo-skeletal function and formulate a plan of action.

INSTRUCTIONS

Utilizing three of your peers or clients in the clinical area, practice inspection and palpation of the muscles, bones and joints and assessment of gait. Remove the Performance Guide cards for Unit 5 from Appendix II. These cards will enable you to practice the skills necessary to meet the Clinical Objectives and complete the Response Sheets. On each Response Sheet you will be expected to (1) ask questions which elicit possible symptoms, (2) systematically describe your findings, (3) localize any abnormalities present and (4) summarize your examination findings using the S.O.A.P. method of recording.

When you have mastered the Clinical Objectives and completed the Response Sheet, arrange to demonstrate your skills to your laboratory instructor or preceptor.

EQUIPMENT

Tape measure

OPTIONAL ACTIVITIES

These films demonstrate techniques of the musculoskeletal examination.
a) Bates: "The Musculoskeletal System" (film).
b) Blue-Hill Educational Systems, Inc.: "Musculo-Skeletal Examination" (a video tape cassette).

RESPONSE SHEET—THE MUSCULOSKELETAL SYSTEM

Client_______________________________

Date_______________________ Age _______ Sex_______

Examiner_______________________________

I. Health History

II. Physical Examination

    A. General Function, Posture and Gait

    B. Head and Neck

    C. Hands and Wrists

    D. Elbows

    E. Shoulders

    F. Feet and Ankles

G. Knees

H. Hips

I. Spine

Summarize your findings using the S.O.A.P. method.

S. (Client's observations, complaints, health history)

O. (Physical findings)

A. (Assessment of problem, data, prognosis)

P. (Plans for further evaluation, care, teaching)

Client_______________________________

Date_____________________ Age________ Sex________

Examiner_______________________________

I. Health History

II. Physical Examination

    A. General Function, Posture and Gait

    B. Head and Neck

    C. Hands and Wrists

    D. Elbows

    E. Shoulders

    F. Feet and Ankles

G. Knees

H. Hips

I. Spine

Summarize your findings using the S.O.A.P. method.

S. (Client's observations, complaints, health history)

O. (Physical findings)

A. (Assessment of problem, data, prognosis)

P. (Plans for further evaluation, care, teaching)

RESPONSE SHEET—THE MUSCULOSKELETAL SYSTEM

Client _______________________________________

Date _________________________ Age ________ Sex ________

Examiner _____________________________________

I. Health History

II. Physical Examination

    A. General Function, Posture and Gait

    B. Head and Neck

    C. Hands and Wrists

    D. Elbows

    E. Shoulders

    F. Feet and Ankles

G. Knees

H. Hips

I. Spine

Summarize your findings using the S.O.A.P. method.

S. (Client's observations, complaints, health history)

O. (Physical findings)

A. (Assessment of problem, data, prognosis)

P. (Plans for further evaluation, care, teaching)

Name_______________________________

Date_______________________________

PRE-TEST

UNIT 6

1. Signs and symptoms which should alert the examiner to possible neurological dysfunction include
    1. decreased hearing ability.
    2. difficulty speaking clearly.
    3. dilated pupils.
    4. disequilibrium.
    5. loss of temperature sense.
    a) 2 and 5 are correct.
    b) 1 and 4 are correct.
    c) 2, 3, 4 and 5 are correct.
    d) 1, 2, 4 and 5 are correct.
    e) all of the above are correct.

Match the following:

2. _______ Lower motor neuron lesion   a) Absent corneal reflex
                                            b) Flaccid paralysis
3. _______ Lesion V cranial nerve   c) Spastic paralysis
                                            d) Facial paralysis
4. _______ Lesion VII cranial nerve   e) Ptosis

5. _______ Upper motor neuron lesion

6. Ocular movement is controlled by
    a) cranial nerve II.
    b) cranial nerves II, III, IV.
    c) cranial nerves III, IV, VI.
    d) cranial nerves IV, V, VI.

7. General cerebral functioning can be assessed by asking the client to
    a) perform rapid alternating movements.
    b) identify objects by touch.
    c) differentiate between warm and cold temperatures.
    d) perform the Romberg test.
    e) demonstrate recall of past, recent or immediate events.

8. To test for patency of the IX and X cranial nerves, the examiner should check
    1. swallowing ability.
    2. strength of trapezius and sternocleidomastoid muscles.
    3. gag reflex.
    4. elevation of the uvula when the palate is stroked.
    a) 1 and 3 are correct.
    b) 1, 3 and 4 are correct.
    c) 2 only is correct.
    d) all of the above are correct.

9. To assess cerebellar functioning the examiner primarily evaluates
   a) proprioception.
   b) muscle coordination.
   c) muscle strength.
   d) deep tendon reflexes.
   e) all of the above.

10. Fine muscle twitchings which often occur with lower motor neuron dysfunction are called
    a) tics.
    b) clonus.
    c) fasciculations.
    d) tremors.
    e) nystagmus.

11. With a lower motor neuron lesion, the client may demonstrate
    1. flaccid paralysis.
    2. tics.
    3. absence of tendon reflexes.
    4. spastic paralysis.
    5. hyperactive tendon reflexes.
    a) 1, 2 and 3 are correct.
    b) 2, 4 and 5 are correct.
    c) 1 and 5 are correct.
    d) 1 and 3 are correct.
    e) 4 and 5 are correct.

12. Stimulation of the triceps muscle elicits
    1. contraction of the biceps muscle.
    2. extension of the forearm.
    3. relaxation of the triceps muscle.
    4. flexion of the forearm.
    5. relaxation of the biceps muscle.
    a) 2 only is correct.
    b) 1, 3 and 4 are correct.
    c) 4 and 5 are correct.
    d) 1 and 2 are correct.
    e) 2 and 5 are correct.

13. Testing the abdominal reflex
    1. is done to assess deep tendon reflexes.
    2. is performed by stroking each quadrant of the abdomen.
    3. normally elicits movement of the umbilicus away from the stimulus.
    4. normally elicits movement of the umbilicus toward the stimulus.
    5. causes the abdominal muscles to contract in the opposite quadrant.
    a) 1, 2, 3 and 5 are correct.
    b) 1, 2, 4 and 5 are correct.
    c) 2, 3 and 5 are correct.
    d) 2 and 4 are correct.
    e) 2 and 5 are correct.

14. Visual acuity is controlled by
    a) cranial nerves III, IV, VI.
    b) cranial nerves II, IV, VI.
    c) cranial nerve II.
    d) cranial nerve VII.
    e) none of the above nerves.

15. The Babinski reflex is
    a) plantar flexion of the foot and fanning of the toes.
    b) an abnormal reflex not normally present in adults.
    c) dorsiflexion of the foot and fanning of the toes.
    d) both a and c.
    e) both b and c.

16. When testing the VIII cranial nerve the examiner should check
    1. Weber test results.
    2. Balance.
    3. Stereognosis.
    4. Palatal reflex.
    5. Tinnitus.
    a) 1, 2 and 3 are correct.
    b) 1, 2 and 5 are correct.
    c) 4 only is correct.
    d) 1 and 5 are correct.
    e) none of the above are correct.

17. Loss of sensation without loss of movement is called
    a) paralysis.
    b) paraplegia.
    c) aphasia.
    d) anesthesia.
    e) apraxia.

18. Assessment of the sensory system includes evaluation of
    1. vibration perception.
    2. Rinne test findings.
    3. temperature perception.
    4. point localization.
    5. sense of smell.
    a) 1, 3 and 5 are correct.
    b) 1, 3 and 4 are correct.
    c) 2 and 5 are correct.
    d) 3 only is correct.
    e) all of the above are correct.

19. A client's inability to shrug the shoulders may indicate abnormality of
    a) cranial nerve XI.
    b) cranial nerve XII.
    c) cranial nerve IX.
    d) none of the above cranial nerves.

20. Lateral deviation of the tongue and lack of tongue strength may indicate abnormality

    of the ________ cranial nerve.
    a) IV
    b) V
    c) XI
    d) XII

Number 6

The Neurological Examination

RATIONALE

The purpose of this self-instructional unit is to help you learn to do a basic neurological assessment. The unit focuses on six areas: mental status, cranial nerves, cerebellar function, motor system, sensory system and reflexes. After completing this unit you will be able to utilize the observational and motor skills necessary to evaluate the integrity of the nervous system.

GLOSSARY OF TERMS

Review the following terms before and after completing this unit. You should be able to define or describe them readily.

Agnosia ____

Agraphia ____

Aphasia ____

Apraxia ____

Clonus ____

Decerebrate posturing ____

Decorticate posturing ____

Dysarthria ____

Dysphagia ____

Extinction phenomenon ____

Fasciculation ____

Flaccidity ____

Lower motor neuron ____

Nystagmus ____

Paresis (hemiparesis, paraparesis,
   quadriparesis) ____

-plegia (monoplegia, hemiplegia, paraplegia) _______________________________

Point localization ____

Proprioception ____

Spasticity ____

Stereognosis ____

Stereotaxis ____

Tic ____

Tremor ____

Two-point discrimination ____

Upper motor neuron ____

COGNITIVE OBJECTIVES

At the end of this unit you will demonstrate knowledge of assessment of the neurological system by your ability to:

1. Describe signs and symptoms of neurological dysfunction.

2. Name and describe the five areas of general cerebral function which are observed during the interview:
   a. General behavior.
   b. Level of consciousness.
   c. Intellectual performance.
   d. Emotional status.
   e. Thought content.

3. Outline the cranial nerves, the tests used to assess their integrity and the normal and abnormal responses.

4. List the functions of the cerebellum and review tests of cerebellar functioning.

5. Describe evaluation of the motor system for
   a. muscle size, tone, strength.
   b. involuntary movements.

6. Describe differences between upper and lower motor neuron dysfunction.

7. List the sensory modalities routinely tested during a neurological assessment (touch, vibration, position, temperature, superficial pain).

8. List the deep tendon reflexes, site of stimulus and normal response.

9. List and describe the superficial reflexes:
   a. Abdominal.
   b. Cremasteric.

10. Describe the following abnormal reflexes:
    a. Babinski.
    b. Chaddock.
    c. Hoffmann.

LEARNING ACTIVITIES

The Learning Activities contain the information necessary for meeting the Cognitive Objectives. Select one and proceed to work with it until you have mastered the material. Use the Cognitive Objectives as a guide for study. A Self-Test is provided so that you can check what you have learned. If you have difficulty with the Self-Test, please review the material in this unit before proceeding to the Clinical Objectives.

Reading Activities

a) Bates: *A Guide to Physical Examination*. Read pp. 263–269 for a discussion of anatomy and physiology (you will not be expected to know specific spinal tracts) and pp. 270–271 for an outline of the cranial nerves. Examination techniques and common abnormal findings are found on pp. 272–305. Numerous drawings aid understanding.

b) DeGowin and DeGowin: *Bedside Diagnostic Examination*, Chapter 11, "The Neurologic Examination," presents the experienced practitioner with in-depth information about all parts of the neurological examination. Examination procedures are well explained. Emphasis is on differentiating abnormalities.

c) Delp and Manning: *Major's Physical Diagnosis*, Chapter 13, "Examination of the Nervous System," presents the principles and procedures for a neurological screening examination. Familiarity with anatomy and physiology is assumed. The discussion of mental status is particularly valuable. More detailed reading in all areas of neurological examination is necessary to meet the objectives.

d) *Essentials of the Neurological Examination*, distributed by the Smith, Kline & French Laboratories. This booklet systematically outlines tests for cerebral function, cranial nerves, cerebellar function, motor and sensory systems and reflexes. Normal and abnormal findings are included. Excellent diagrams aid understanding.

e) Gillies and Alyn: *Patient Assessment and Management by the Nurse Practitioner*, "The Neurologic Examination," presents broad coverage of procedures, techniques and normal findings. Does not differentiate between upper and lower motor neuron dysfunction. Abnormal findings are not generally included.

f) Judge and Zuidema: *Methods of Clinical Examination: A Physiologic Approach*, Chapter 20, "Nervous System," covers the basics of neurological examination in varying degrees of detail. Use your study guide to ascertain where additional reading is needed. Testing of the cranial nerves is clearly presented. The glossary at the beginning of the chapter is very helpful.

g) Prior and Silberstein: *Physical Diagnosis*, Chapter 15, "Nervous System." This chapter presents a comprehensive discussion of cerebral function, cranial nerves, cerebellar function, motor and sensory systems and reflexes. Lower motor neuron dysfunctions are described in detail. The emphasis is on normal examination findings.

h) Sana and Judge: *Physical Appraisal Methods in Nursing Practice*, Chapter 13, "Detection of Alterations in Neuromuscular Functioning." This chapter begins with an informative glossary which is followed by a comprehensive discussion of the neurological examination with emphasis on normal findings. Symptoms of central nervous system dysfunction are discussed, providing a well-rounded approach.

i) Sherman and Fields: *Guide to Patient Evaluation*, Chapter 18, "The Neurologic Examination." This reading presents a clear and systematic overview of the neurological examination. An excellent starting point for the novice or as a review for the experienced practitioner.

Audiovisual Activities

a) Blue-Hill Educational Systems, Inc.: "The Neurologic Examination" (video tape No. 17). The first part of this lecture deals with assessment of mental status. It then continues with evaluation of cranial nerves, motor and sensory systems. A detailed evaluation of muscles, reflexes and coordination is presented.

Supplemental Activity

a) Plum and Posner: *Diagnosis of Stupor and Coma*, 2nd ed.

SELF-TEST

This Self-Test is for you. Use it to check how well you have learned the material presented in this unit. The answers follow the test.

1. Symptoms which should alert the examiner to possible neurological dysfunction include
    1. severe mood swings.
    2. slurred speech.
    3. presence of corneal reflex.
    4. absence of Babinski reflex.
    5. poor motor coordination.
   a) 2 and 5 are correct.
   b) 3 and 4 are correct.
   c) 1, 2, 3 and 5 are correct.
   d) 1, 2 and 5 are correct.
   e) all of the above are correct.

2. The levels of consciousness range from alert to
   a) confusion.
   b) delirium.
   c) stupor.
   d) coma.

3. Disease of the III cranial nerve may result in
    1. inability to look nasally downward.
    2. ptosis.
    3. absence of corneal reflex.

    4. eyes deviated temporally downward.
    5. pupillary dilatation.
a) 1 only is correct.
b) 3 and 5 are correct.
c) 2, 4 and 5 are correct.
d) 2, 3 and 4 are correct.
e) none of the above are correct.

4. Asking the client to repeat a series of numbers backward is done primarily to test
a) cerebellar function.
b) sensorium and intellectual resources.
c) for agraphia.
d) memory for past events.

5. The ability to swallow is a test for patency of the ________ cranial nerve.
a) VI
b) VIII
c) IX
d) X
e) XII

6. Having the client shrug both shoulders against resistance tests
    1. strength of triceps muscle.
    2. XI cranial nerve patency.
    3. strength of the trapezius muscle.
    4. X cranial nerve patency.
    5. XII cranial nerve patency.
a) 2 and 3 are correct.
b) 1 and 4 are correct.
c) 4 only is correct.
d) 2, 3 and 5 are correct.
e) none of the above are correct.

7. The primary functions of the cerebellum are
    1. muscle strength.
    2. proprioception.
    3. balance.
    4. muscle coordination.
a) 2, 3 and 4 are correct.
b) 3 and 4 are correct.
c) 1, 3 and 4 are correct.
d) 4 only is correct.
e) all of the above are correct.

8. Fine visible twitching movements of a bundle of muscle is
    1. a tic.
    2. called fasciculation.
    3. frequently associated with lower motor neuron dysfunction.
    4. a sign of cerebellar disease.
a) 1 only is correct.
b) 1 and 4 are correct.
c) 2 and 3 are correct.
d) 2, 3 and 4 are correct.
e) 1, 3 and 4 are correct.

9. With an *upper* motor neuron lesion, the client may demonstrate
   1. flaccid paralysis.
   2. tics.
   3. hypoactive tendon reflexes.
   4. spastic paralysis.
   5. clonus.
   a) 4 and 5 are correct.
   b) 1, 2 and 3 are correct.
   c) 1 and 3 are correct.
   d) 4 only is correct.
   e) none of the above are correct.

10. Assessment of the sensory system includes evaluation of
    1. vibration perception.
    2. stereognosis.
    3. deep pain.
    4. point localization.
    5. parallel points on opposite sides of the body.
    a) 1 and 5 are correct.
    b) 2, 3 and 4 are correct.
    c) 1, 2, 4 and 5 are correct.
    d) all of the above are correct.

11. Stimulation of the biceps tendon elicits
    1. contraction of the biceps muscle.
    2. extension of the forearm.
    3. relaxation of the triceps muscle.
    4. flexion of the forearm.
    a) 1, 2 and 3 are correct.
    b) 1, 3 and 4 are correct.
    c) 1 and 4 are correct.
    d) 2 and 3 are correct.

12. In testing the normal abdominal reflex
    1. the abdomen is stroked toward the umbilicus.
    2. the umbilicus moves toward the area stroked.
    3. the abdomen is stroked away from the umbilicus.
    4. the umbilicus moves away from the area stroked.
    a) 1 and 4 are correct.
    b) 2 and 3 are correct.
    c) 1 and 2 are correct.
    d) 3 and 4 are correct.

13. The Babinski reflex is
    1. plantar flexion of the foot and fanning of the toes.
    2. a superficial reflex.
    3. normally present in adults.
    4. dorsiflexion of the foot and fanning of the toes.
    a) 1 only is correct.
    b) 1, 2 and 3 are correct.
    c) 4 only is correct.
    d) 3 and 4 are correct.
    e) 1 and 2 are correct.

SELF-TEST KEY

1. (d) Severe mood swings, slurred speech and poor motor coordination are signs of cerebral, cranial nerve and cerebellar dysfunction, respectively. Normally the corneal reflex is present. Presence of the Babinski reflex is an abnormal finding in adults, indicating upper motor neuron dysfunction.

2. (d) The deepest state of unconsciousness is coma, in which the client is unresponsive to any stimuli and reflexes are absent. Confusion means impaired perception and defective memory. Delirium refers to confusion associated with hallucinations. Stupor is a somnolent state in which the client responds to painful stimuli and reflexes are intact.

3. (c) With paralysis of the III cranial nerve, only the IV and VI cranial nerves are left to innervate the eye muscles. Since the IV directs the eye down and nasally and the VI directs the eye horizontal and temporally, the eye assumes a midway position (temporally and down). Ptosis of the lid and a dilated, nonreactive pupil also occur with III nerve damage. The corneal reflex is mediated by the V cranial nerve.

4. (b) Cerebellar functions are concerned with balance and coordination. Agraphia is the inability to write. Memory for past events is usually determined during history taking. The ability to repeat a series of numbers backward demonstrates a clear sensorium, memory for recent events and good intellectual performance.

5. (d) The VI cranial nerve mediates eye movements. The VIII mediates hearing and balance. Although the IX and X cranial nerves are usually tested together, it is the X cranial nerve which makes swallowing possible. The XII cranial nerve mediates movements of the tongue.

6. (a) The triceps muscle would be tested by extension of the forearm against resistance. The XI cranial nerve innervates the trapezius and sternocleidomastoid muscles. The X cranial nerve supplies motor fibers to the pharynx, larynx and soft palate. The XII supplies motor fibers to the tongue.

7. (b) The cerebellum controls balance and coordination. Muscle strength depends on both musculoskeletal and neurological factors. Proprioception is the ability to sense body movement and position.

8. (c) Fasciculations result from lower motor neuron dysfunctions in which the basic reflex arc is absent, but stimulatory impulses are still coming from the brain to innervate individual muscle bundles. A tic is a spasmodic twitch usually associated with nervous habits.

9. (a) A spastic rather than flaccid paralysis results from upper motor neuron dysfunction because the basic reflex arc is still intact; additionally, this tends to make the tendon reflex hyperactive, as is demonstrated by the presence of clonus.

10. (c) Deep pain sense is only tested in special cases as in evaluation of coma. Assessment of the sensory system usually covers superficial tactile, superficial pain, vibration, temperature and position senses. The ability to distinguish two-point discrimination, point localization, stereognosis and extinction phenomenon may also be tested.

11. (b) Stretch of the biceps tendon causes a reflex shortening of the biceps muscle. This contraction flexes the forearm. A reciprocal relaxation of the triceps muscle occurs simultaneously.

12. (c) The superficial abdominal reflex is performed by stroking the abdomen, in each of the four quadrants, from the periphery toward the umbilicus. The abdominal muscles contract so that the umbilicus moves toward the stimulus. An abnormal response indicates neurological damage at or above cranial nerve VII, VIII or IX.

13. (c) The Babinski reflex is a pathological reflex when found in adults and demonstrates an extensor movement of the foot and toes.

CLINICAL COMPONENT

Having completed the cognitive portion of this unit, you are now ready to proceed to the Clinical Objectives. The purpose of the Clinical Component is to assess the neurological system for normal function and to detect the presence, location and extent of any dysfunction.

CLINICAL OBJECTIVES

At the end of this unit you will perform assessment of the neurological system correlating physical examination skills and physiological principles. You will be able to:

1. Demonstrate knowledge of signs and symptoms of neurological dysfunction by obtaining a pertinent health history.

2. Make observations and ask questions which elicit information about cerebral functioning.
   a. general behavior
   b. level of consciousness
   c. intellectual performance
   d. emotional status
   e. thought content

3. Test for patency of the twelve cranial nerves.

4. Demonstrate at least three tests of cerebellar functioning.

5. Evaluate the motor system by systematically testing muscle size, tone, strength and involuntary movements.

6. Differentiate between signs of upper and lower motor neuron dysfunction.

7. Employ at least five tests for sensory modalities: touch, vibration, position, temperature and superficial pain.

8. Demonstrate evaluation of deep tendon, superficial and abnormal reflexes.

9. Utilize the S.O.A.P. method of recording to systematically describe your findings, make an assessment regarding normality and formulate a plan of action.

INSTRUCTIONS

Utilizing three of your peers or clients in the clinical area, practice assessment of the neurological system. Remove the Performance Guide cards for Unit 6 from Appendix II. These cards will enable you to practice the skills necessary to meet the Clinical Objectives and complete the Response Sheets. On each Response Sheet you will be expected to (1) ask questions which elicit possible symptoms; (2) systematically describe your examination findings; (3) localize any abnormalities if they are present; and (4) summarize the examination using the S.O.A.P. method.

When you have mastered the Clinical Objectives and completed the Response Sheets arrange to demonstrate your skills to your laboratory instructor or preceptor.

EQUIPMENT

Common condiments for testing taste and smell senses (e.g., salt, sugar, coffee, cloves)
Cotton ball
Pin
Reflex hammer
Small flashlight
Tongue blades
Tuning fork

Optional Activities

These films demonstrate techniques of neurological assessment.
a) Bates: "Neurologic Examination – Parts I and II" (film).
b) Blue-Hill Educational Systems, Inc.: "Neurological Examination" (55-minute video tape cassette).

RESPONSE SHEET — THE NEUROLOGICAL EXAMINATION

Client _______________________________

Date _________________ Age _______ Sex _______

Examiner _____________________________

I. Health History

II. Physical Examination

   A. General Cerebral

   B. Cranial Nerves

      1. I

      2. II

      3. III, IV, VI

      4. V

      5. VII

      6. VIII

      7. IX, X

      8. XI

      9. XII

   C. Cerebellar

D. Motor System

E. Sensory System

F. Reflexes

	Bi	Tri	BR	P	A	Pl (↑/↓)	Abd	Cre	Bab	Hoff	Jaw
L											
R											

0 = absent;   + = hypoactive;   ++ = normal;   +++ = hyperactive;   ++++ = clonus
↑ dorsiflexion; ↓ plantar flexion

Summarize your findings using S.O.A.P. method.

S. **(Client's observations, complaints, health history)**

O. **(Physical findings)**

A. **(Assessment of the problem, data, prognosis)**

P. **(Plans for further evaluation, care, teaching)**

RESPONSE SHEET — THE NEUROLOGICAL EXAMINATION

Client ____

Date ___________________________ Age _________ Sex _________

Examiner ____

I. **Health History**

II. **Physical Examination**

   A. **General Cerebral**

   B. **Cranial Nerves**

     1. I

     2. II

     3. III, IV, VI

     4. V

     5. VII

     6. VIII

     7. IX, X

     8. XI

     9. XII

   C. **Cerebellar**

D. Motor System

E. Sensory System

F. Reflexes

	Bi	Tri	BR	P	A	Pl ($\uparrow$/$\downarrow$)	Abd	Cre	Bab	Hoff	Jaw
L											
R											

0 = absent; + = hypoactive; ++ = normal; +++ = hyperactive; ++++ = clonus
$\uparrow$ dorsiflexion; $\downarrow$ plantar flexion

Summarize your findings using S.O.A.P. method.

S. (Client's observations, complaints, health history)

O. (Physical findings)

A. (Assessment of the problem, data, prognosis)

P. (Plans for further evaluation, care, teaching)

RESPONSE SHEET — THE NEUROLOGICAL EXAMINATION

Client ____

Date _________________________ Age _______ Sex _______

Examiner ____

I. Health History

II. Physical Examination

    A. General Cerebral

    B. Cranial Nerves

        1. I

        2. II

        3. III, IV, VI

        4. V

        5. VII

        6. VIII

        7. IX, X

        8. XI

        9. XII

    C. Cerebellar

D. Motor System

E. Sensory System

F. Reflexes

	Bi	Tri	BR	P	A	Pl (↑/↓)	Abd	Cre	Bab	Hoff	Jaw
L											
R											

0 = absent; + = hypoactive;   ++ = normal;   +++ = hyperactive;   ++++ = clonus
↑ dorsiflexion; ↓ plantar flexion

Summarize your findings using S.O.A.P. method.

S. (Client's observations, complaints, health history)

O. (Physical findings)

A. (Assessment of the problem, data, prognosis)

P. (Plans for further evaluation, care, teaching)

SECTION II

HEAD AND NECK

PRE-TEST

UNIT 7

Match the following columns:

1. __*b*__ Drooping of the eyelid

2. __*E*__ "Bulging" eyeballs

3. __*A*__ Near-sightedness

a) Myopia
b) Ptosis
c) Lid lag
d) Enophthalmos
e) Exophthalmos

4. The conjunctiva covers
   a) both the insides of the eyelids and the sclera.
   b) only the eyeball.
   c) only the insides of the eyelids.
   d) both the insides of the eyelids and the cornea.

5. The iris is examined for color and integrity.
   a) True
   b) False

6. Mr. Abbey wears glasses for reading only. His right eye is tested for visual acuity with the Snellen chart 20 ft away. He reads row 30 correctly. The written result would be
   a) 20/30 with correction.
   b) 30/20 OS with correction.
   c) 20/30 OD with correction.
   d) 20/30 OD without correction.
   e) none of the above.

7. An abnormal fleshy growth which grows in a horizontal band over the cornea is called
   a) chalazion.
   b) blepharitis.
   c) pterygium.
   d) hordeolum.

8. Eye movements are controlled by the __________ cranial nerves.
   a) II, III
   b) III, IV, V
   c) IX, X
   d) III, IV, VI

9. Astigmatism refers to
   a) defective curvature of the eye so that images are not sharply focused on the retina.
   b) a muscular defect resulting in uncoordinated eye movements.
   c) rapid, jerky eye movements.
   d) a progressive tendency toward far-sightedness with age.

10. Pupillary reflex is tested by shining a light into one eye and observing
    a) dilation of the pupil directly stimulated and constriction of the other eye.
    b) direct constriction of that eye and consensual dilation of the other pupil.
    c) constriction of that pupil and consensual constriction of the pupil not directly stimulated.
    d) dilation of both pupils.

11. Bilateral exophthalmos may be produced by
    a) increased intraocular pressure.
    b) ptosis of the eyelid.
    c) dehydration.
    d) formation of a chalazion.

12. Accommodation refers to
    1. pupillary constriction when looking at a near object.
    2. pupillary constriction when looking at a far object.
    3. pupillary dilation when looking at a near object.
    4. pupillary dilation when looking at a far object.
    a) 2 only is correct.
    b) 2 and 3 are correct.
    c) 1 and 4 are correct.
    d) 4 only is correct.

13. The ability to look cross-eyed is
    a) convexion.
    b) convergence.
    c) astigmatism.
    d) accommodation.

14. A dull reflection on the cornea when illuminated by light indicates
    a) scarring or ulceration.
    b) normal pigmentation.
    c) increased intraocular pressure.
    d) lid lag.

15. The following structures are *not* observed in examination of the external eye
    1. Cornea
    2. Pupil
    3. Conjunctiva
    4. Sclera
    5. Lacrimal ducts
    6. Posterior chamber
    7. Retina
    a) 2, 4 and 6 are correct.
    b) 1, 5 and 6 are correct.
    c) 6 only is correct.
    d) 6 and 7 are correct.

16. Strabismus is detected by
    a) high tonometry readings.
    b) eye movement during the cover test.
    c) inability to read the Snellen chart with both eyes uncovered.
    d) pupillary dilation when looking at far objects.

Observe the following diagram for questions 17 through 20. Choose the *one* correct abnormality which would result from a lesion in that location.

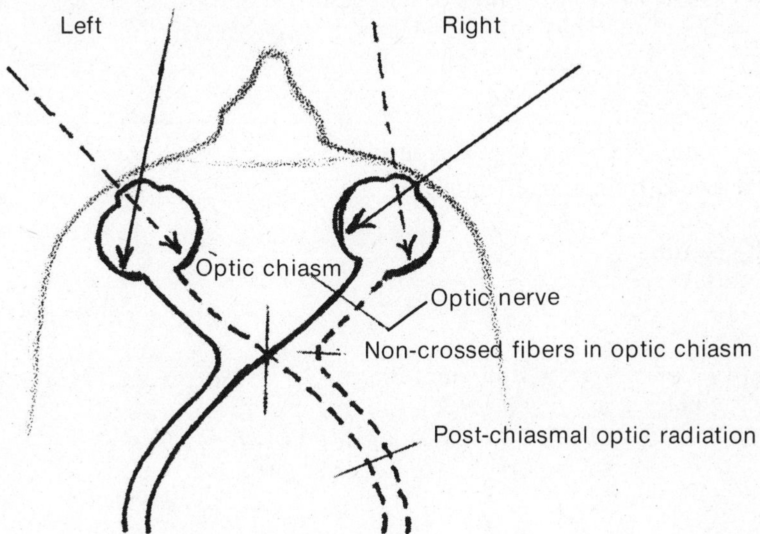

17. A lesion in the optic nerve would produce
    a) homonymous hemianopsia.
    b) unilateral temporal hemianopsia.
    c) unilateral blindness O.D.
    d) unilateral blindness O.S.

18. A lesion in the optic chiasm would produce
    a) bitemporal hemianopsia.
    b) homonymous hemianopsia.
    c) binasal hemianopsia.
    d) total blindness.

19. A lesion in the noncrossed fibers in the optic chiasm causes
    a) unilateral temporal hemianopsia.
    b) unilateral blindness.
    c) unilateral nasal hemianopsia.
    d) homonymous hemianopsia.

20. A lesion in the postchiasmal optic radiation produces
    a) unilateral blindness.
    b) bitemporal hemianopsia.
    c) binasal hemianopsia.
    d) homonymous hemianopsia.

Number 7

Examination of the External Eye

RATIONALE

The purpose of this self-instructional unit is to help you learn inspection and palpation of the external eye. This unit concentrates on the examination of the external structures of the eye and some abnormal findings associated with each of these areas. Visual acuity and examination of the visual fields are also included. After completing this unit, you will be able to evaluate the structures of the external eye, detect and describe an abnormality, test for visual acuity and determine weakness or paralysis of eye muscles.

GLOSSARY OF TERMS

Review the following terms before and after completing this unit. You should be able to define or describe them readily.

Accommodation *adaptation or adjustment of an organ*

Arcus senilis (corneal arcus) *an opaque ring at edge of cornea, seen in middle and especially old age.*

Argyll Robertson pupil *a pupil which constricts on accomodation but not to light*

Astigmatism *defect of vision which results from irregularity in the one or more reffactive structure, cornea.*

Bitemporal hemianopsia *loss of vision in one half of visual field on both sides of temple*

Blepharitis *inflammation of the eyelids*

Cataract *partial or comple opacity of the crystalline lens or its capsule*

Chalazion *tumor of the eyelid from retained secretion of the tarsal glands*

Concave *possessing a curved, depressed surface*

Conjunctivitis *inflammation of the conjunctive*

Convergence *inclination or direction toward a common point*

Convex *rounded*

Diplopia *a disorder of sight in which one object is perceived as two, double vision.*

Enophthalmos _Recession of the eyeball into the orbit._

Entropion _Inversion of the eyelid_

Exophthalmos (proptosis) _Abnormal protrusion of the eyeball_

Ectropion _Eversion of the eyelid_

Hemianopsia _Blindness in one half of visual field: bilateral, unilateral_

Hordeolum _furuncular inflammation of connective tissue of eyelids, near to hair follicle_

Hyperopia _refractive error, suspended accommodation_

Lid lag _lagging of upper lid behind eyeball when pt looks down_

Miosis _abnormal constriction of pupil_

Mydriasis _______________

Myopia _nearsightedness (longer → eyeball)_

Nystagmus _An oscillatory movement of the eyeballs_

Presbyopia _______________

Pterygium _triangular patch of mucous membrane growing on conjunctiva_

Ptosis _drooping of upper eyelid from 3rd cranial nerve damage_

Strabismus _visual axes do not meet at desired objective point_

Visual acuity _measured central vision_

Xanthelasma _Yellowish raised plaque occurring around the eyelid_

COGNITIVE OBJECTIVES

At the end of this unit you will demonstrate knowledge of inspection and palpation of the external eye and visual tests by your ability to:

1. Systematically describe the normal appearance of the external eye structures; list two commonly observed abnormalities for each: lids, lacrimal ducts, conjunctiva, sclera, cornea, iris, pupils.

2. Explain the use of the Snellen chart for testing visual acuity.

3. Describe normal pupillary reactions: direct and consensual constriction, accommodation.

4. Describe the method for gross inspection of the visual fields; relate abnormal findings in the visual field to position of lesions in the optic tract.

5. List the three cranial nerves which innervate eye muscles.
    a. Describe tests for extraocular movement, convergence and stabismus (cover test).
    b. Differentiate between normal and abnormal findings.

LEARNING ACTIVITIES

The Learning Activities contain the information necessary for meeting the Cognitive Objectives. Select one and proceed to work with it until you have mastered the material. Use the Cognitive Objectives as a guide for study. A Self-Test is provided so that you can check how much you know. If you have difficulty with the Self-Test, please review the material in this unit.

Reading Activities

a) Bates: *A Guide to Physical Examination*, Chapter 4, "The Head and Neck," discusses anatomy of the eye, techniques of examination of the external structures, pupillary reactions, visual acuity and visual fields. Common abnormalities are also discussed. Tests for strabismus are very well covered in the chapter on pediatric examination. There are excellent drawings throughout.

b) DeGowin and DeGowin: *Bedside Diagnostic Examination*, pp. 65–100. Valuable for the advanced practitioner or as a reference to supplement more basic readings. Detailed information on all aspects of the examination.

c) Delp and Manning: *Major's Physical Diagnosis*, Chapter 7, provides extensive coverage of abnormalities. Testing procedures are briefly discussed. There are good photographs of abnormal findings. Supplement your reading.

d) Gillies and Alyn: *Patient Assessment and Management by the Nurse Practitioner*, "Examination of the Head and Neck" (pp. 42–46). This section discusses assessment of the external eye, use of the Snellen chart, pupillary reactions and extraocular movements. The cover test and examination of visual fields with related abnormal findings are not included.

e) Judge and Zuidema: *Methods of Clinical Examination: A Physiologic Approach*, Chapter 6, "The Eye" (pp. 61–68, 72–76, 79). Knowledge of anatomy is assumed. Measurement of visual acuity, assessment of ocular movements, inspection of the external structures and testing of pupillary reactions are presented. The chapter also includes a helpful glossary of terms. The cover test for strabismus and assessment of visual fields are not covered.

f) Prior and Silberstein: *Physical Diagnosis*, Chapter 7, "Eyes" (pp. 78–96). This chapter provides clear, comprehensive coverage of all aspects of examination of the external eye.

g) Sana and Judge: *Physical Appraisal Methods in Nursing Practice* (pp. 105–117). This section contains a glossary of pertinent terms. Knowledge of anatomy and physiology is assumed. Procedures are covered in a cursory manner with emphasis on normal findings. Testing of visual acuity is very well done.

h) Sherman and Fields: *Guide to Patient Evaluation* (pp. 72–90). Anatomy and physiology, examination procedures and common abnormal findings are presented in an easy-to-follow manner.

i) Mechner, Francis: "Examination of the Eye—Part I." *AJN*, Vol. 74, No. 11, November 1974. Programmed instruction covers assessment of the external eye structures and offers excellent color photographs. This article does not include any procedural techniques except for tonometry. A good adjunct to any of the reading activities.

Audiovisual Activities

a) Blue-Hill Educational Systems, Inc.: "Eyes 4A and 4B," video tape. (Disregard information on the ophthalmoscopic examination.) This program presents a comprehensive approach to inspection and palpation of the external eye structures. Abnormal findings are described in detail. Visual acuity and use of the Snellen chart are described, as are testing of visual fields and implications of abnormal findings.

b) Concept Media: "The Eye," film strip.

Supplemental Activities

a) Abbott Laboratory Atlas: *Some Pathological Conditions of the Eye, Ear and Throat* contains excellent color photographs to aid in learning.

b) "Diseases of the Eye," Clinical Symposium Reprints. CIBA Pharmaceutical Co.

SELF-TEST

This Self-Test is for you. Use it to check how well you have learned the material presented in the unit. The answers follow the test.

1. Describe the characteristics of each structure observed during examination of the external eye.

    a) lids-

    b) lacrimal ducts-

    c) conjunctiva-

    d) sclera-

    e) cornea

    f) iris-

    g) pupils-

2. A painful red swelling of an eyelash hair follicle is called
    a) chalazion.
    b) blepharitis.
    c) pterygium.
    d) hordeolum.
    e) carcinoma.

3. Visual acuity is tested using the Snellen chart. Briefly explain what 20/20 means.

4. Explain the difference between direct and consensual constriction when testing pupillary reflex.

① It shone directly on eye
② Pupil reacts even though lt not shown on it.

5. Accommodation may be tested by having the client focus on a distant object and then look at an object approximately 6 inches away. At this distance you could expect the pupils to (dilate/constrict).

Constrict

6. Examine the illustration below. For labels a through e, name the place in the optic tract and the abnormality in the visual field that will result from lesions in those areas.

a) *optic nerve damage*
unilateral blindness

b) *optic chiasm*
bitemporal hemianopsia

c) *optic chiasm*
unilateral nasal hemianopsia

d) *post chiasm*
left homonymous hemianopsia

e)

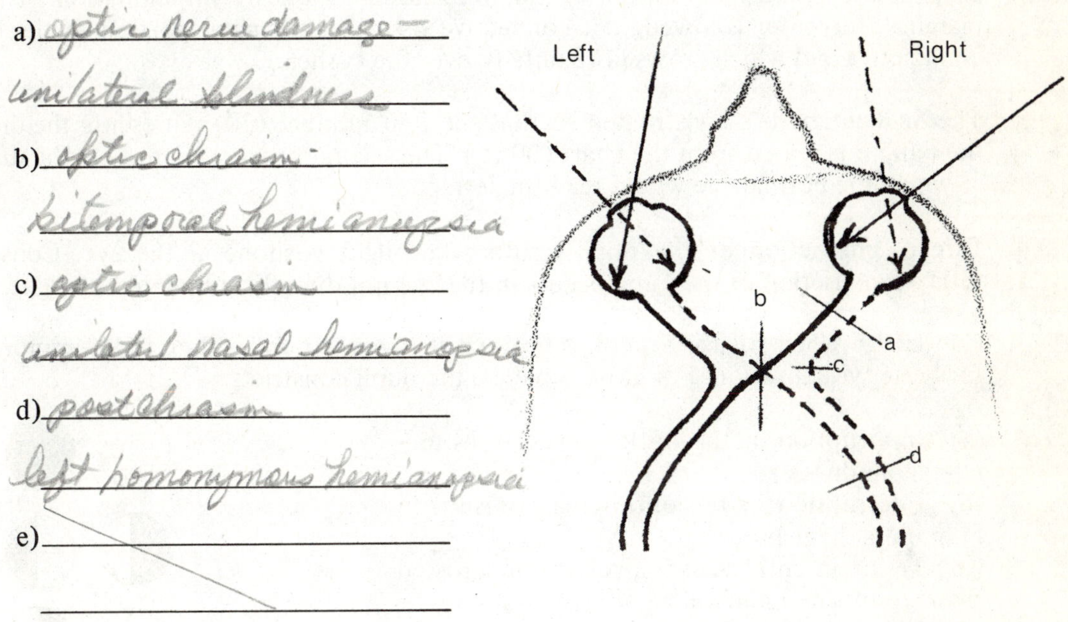

7. List the six cardinal positions of gaze.

a) *horizontal temporal*

b) *up & temporal*

c) *up and nasal*

d) *horizontal nasal*

e) *down & temporal*

f) *down & nasal*

8. Describe the cover test for strabismus.

9. The inability to clearly see far objects is called
   a) hyperopia.
   b) astigmatism.
   c) myopia.
   d) cataract.

SELF-TEST KEY

1. (a) Lids – swelling, lesions, color, direction of lashes, height of pelpebral fissure, blinking.
(b) Ducts – patency, tearing, inflammation.
(c) Conjunctiva – vascularity, lesions.
(d) Sclera – color.
(e) Cornea – depth of anterior chamber, curvature, opacities.
(f) Iris – color, integrity.
(g) Pupils – size, shape, symmetry, direct/consensual reaction to light, accommodation.

2. (d) A hordeolum, or sty, is an infection at the base of an eyelash follicle. Chalazion is a painless cystlike mass of the eyelid. Blepharitis is a scaly inflammation of the lid margin. Pterygium is a wedge of connective tissue on the nasal portion of the bulbar conjunctiva and which grows horizontally over the cornea.

3. The Snellen chart is constructed so that the first number (20) represents the distance the patient is seated from the chart (20 ft.). The second number represents the distance at which the normal eye would read the letters.

4. Direct constriction of the pupil results when light is shone at the eye. Consensual reflex constriction of the pupil occurs in the eye not directly stimulated by light.

5. Constrict. When focusing on objects at a distance, the pupils dilate to let in more light for better visualization. For closer objects, the pupil constricts.

6. (a) Interruption in the optic nerve causes unilateral blindness.
(b) Interruption in the optic chiasm results in bitemporal hemianopsia.
(c) Lesion in optic chiasm involving noncrossed fibers results in unilateral nasal hemianopsia.
(d) Lesion in the postchiasmal optic radiation results in left homonymous hemianopsia.

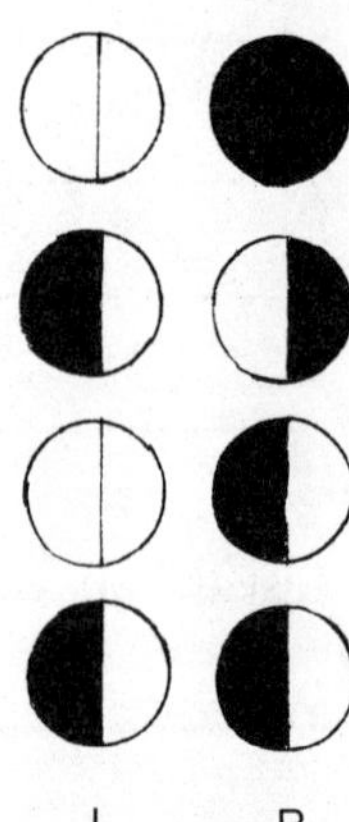

7. (a) Horizontal temporal
(b) Up and temporal
(c) Up and nasal
(d) Horizontal nasal
(e) Down and nasal
(f) Down and temporal

8. To detect ocular muscle weakness and resultant pupil deviation, the examiner directs the client to look straight ahead at an object at least 6 ft away, then covers one eye and observes for movement in the uncovered eye, uncovers the eye and looks for movement in both eyes. If one or both move, strabismus is present. (Repeat for other eye.)

9. (c) Myopia, or near-sightedness, means that far objects are not clearly distinguished. Astigmatism is due to an abnormal curvature of the lens so that a ray of light is not

sharply focused on the retina. A cataract is an opacity, frequently on the cornea, which will distort vision at any distance.

CLINICAL COMPONENT

The Clinical Component for Units 7 through 11 is presented at the end of this section in Unit 12, Head and Neck: Clinical Component (see p. 217). Preview the Clinical Objectives in Unit 12 and the Performance Guide cards for Unit 12 in Appendix II. Facilitate your learning by practicing these skills before proceeding to the next unit.

UNIT 8

1. The optic disc
   1. normally has a regular shape and indistinct margins.
   2. has a cup:disc ratio which is normally greater than 1:2.
   3. usually is darker pink than the general background.
   4. scleral crescent is a normal variation.
   5. is located on the temporal side of the fundus.
   a) 1 and 5 are correct.
   b) 3 and 4 are correct.
   c) 2 and 4 are correct.
   d) 1, 2, 3 and 5 are correct.
   e) none of the above are correct.

2. The general background
   1. is examined for pigmentation and integrity.
   2. pigmentation generally corresponds to the skin tones of the individual.
   3. may contain drusen, an indication of serious eye disease in the elderly.
   4. always shows a vascular choroidal pattern.
   a) 1 and 2 are correct.
   b) 3 and 4 are correct.
   c) 1 and 3 are correct.
   d) 2 and 4 are correct.
   e) all of the above are correct.

3. The retinal vessels
   1. narrow as they approach the periphery.
   2. have an AV ratio which is normally less than 1:2.
   3. may have constrictions as normal variants.
   4. have AV crossings that always result in backup of venous blood.
   5. normally the veins reflect a narrow white stripe.
   a) 1 and 2 are correct.
   b) 1 only is correct.
   c) 3 and 4 are correct.
   d) 2 and 5 are correct.
   e) none of the above are correct.

4. The macular region
   1. includes the fovea as a dark pit in the center.
   2. is a highly vascular area.
   3. is examined for pigment distribution and hemorrhage.
   4. is located to the nasal side of the fundus.
   a) 2 only is correct.
   b) 2 and 4 are correct.
   c) 1, 3 and 4 are correct.
   d) 1 and 3 are correct.
   e) none of the above are correct.

5. A dark shadow against the fundus glow (red reflex) indicates
   a) hemorrhage.
   b) glaucoma.
   c) opacity.
   d) a normal finding.
   e) none of the above.

6. Death of the optic nerve (optic atrophy) would show
   a) an enlarged cup.
   b) a hyperemic disc.
   c) a yellowish disc.
   d) a pale disc.
   e) a normal cup and disc.

7. The red numbers on the ophthalmoscope
   1. are called diopters.
   2. have a longer focal length than the black numbers.
   3. are used to see the more superficial parts of the internal eye.
   4. are used routinely when checking for corneal opacities.
   a) 1 and 4 are correct.
   b) 1 and 2 are correct.
   c) 2 and 3 are correct.
   d) 2 and 4 are correct.
   e) 1 and 3 are correct.

8. The small, round white light on the ophthalmoscope is used for examining the client with
   a) dilated pupils.
   b) constricted pupils.

9. An increased cup:disc ratio should make you suspect
   a) glaucoma.
   b) retinal hemorrhage.
   c) a normal variant.
   d) papilledema.

10. Increased intraocular pressure
    1. is determined by palpation.
    2. is indicated by a "boggy" eyeball
    3. may indicate advanced glaucoma.
    4. results from dehydration.
    a) 1 and 2 are correct.
    b) 2 and 4 are correct.
    c) 2 and 3 are correct.
    d) 1 and 3 are correct.

11. Engorgement and swelling of the optic disc due to venous stasis is
    a) papilledema.
    b) vitreous opacity.
    c) glaucoma.
    d) all of the above.

Match the examination findings in items 12 through 16 with the area where each would be seen.

12. __*D*__ Avascular area

13. __*A*__ Physiological cup

14. __*C*__ Cotton-wool area

15. __*B*__ Dot hemorrhage

16. ______ AV crossing

a) Disc
b) Vessels
c) General background
d) Macula

17. Hemorrhages in the superficial layers of the retina appear as
    a) dots or blots.
    b) solid patches.
    c) flame-shaped or linear markings.
    d) white crescents.

18. When eliciting the red reflex, a corneal opacity appears to
    a) move in the same direction.
    b) remain stationary.
    c) moves in the opposite direction.
    d) is variable in different clients.

19. The correct procedure for checking for opacities includes
    1. using your right eye to examine client's right eye.
    2. using a semidark room.
    3. a minus diopter setting.
    4. approaching the client directly in his or her line of view.
    a) 1, 2 and 4 are correct.
    b) 1, 2 and 3 are correct.
    c) 3 only is correct.
    d) 2 and 4 are correct.
    e) all of the above are correct.

20. Exudates are
    1. yellowish
    2. flat.
    3. white.
    4. fluffy.
    5. red.
    a) 1 and 2 are correct.
    b) 2 and 5 are correct.
    c) 3 and 4 are correct.
    d) 1 and 4 are correct.
    e) 2 and 3 are correct.

Number 8

The Ophthalmoscopic Examination

RATIONALE

This self-instructional unit is designed to help you learn how to use the ophthalmoscope to distinguish normal from abnormal findings in the internal eye. The unit concentrates on the technique of handling the ophthalmoscope and examination of the fundus. After completing the unit, you will be able to utilize the ophthalmoscope to visualize and describe the disc, vessels, general background and macula; locate opacities; and make judgments regarding normality.

GLOSSARY OF TERMS

Review the following terms before and after completing this unit. You should be able to define or describe them readily.

AV crossings (nicking) *localized constriction of retinal veins*

Cataract *partial or complete opacity of crystalline lens*

Copper wiring _______________

Cotton-wool areas *white areas of degenerated retinal elements & leukocytes (hyper tension)*

Cup:disc ratio _______________

Diopter *unit of measurement of the refractive power of an optic lens*

Drusen *colloidal excrescences*

Exudate *material c̄ high protein & cell content that has passed thru vessel wall into tissue*

Fovea *small pit or depression, most sensitive pt of vision*

Glaucoma *increase in intraocular pressure → hardness of globe*

Hyperemia *increased blood in a part, resulting in distention of vessel*

Macula *spot (yellowish) on retina*

Microaneurysm *aneurysmal dilation of a capillary*

Optic atrophy *atrophy of optic nerve*

Optic disc *circular area or retina, site of convergence of fibers to form optic nerve*

OD *Right eye*

OS *left eye*

Papilledema *edema of the optic disc*

Red reflex *red glow of lt seen to emerge from the pupil when the interior of the eye is illuminated*

COGNITIVE OBJECTIVES

At the end of this unit you will demonstrate knowledge of the ophthalmoscopic examination by your ability to:

1. Describe the location of the disc, vessels and macula in the left and right eye.

2. Systematically describe characteristics and normal variants of the fundus.
   a. Disc: shape and margins, color, cup:disc ratio; scleral or pigmented crescents.
   b. Vessels: relative width of arteries and veins, regularity of the blood column, AV crossings.
   c. Background: pigmentation, choroidal pattern; drusen.
   d. Macula: pigmentation, integrity.

3. Discuss the physiological basis and clinical implications of abnormal findings in the fundus.
   a. Disc: blurred margins, optic atrophy, hyperemia, cup:disc ratio greater than 1:2, asymmetry.
   b. Vessels: generalized narrowing, AV ratio less than 1:2, constrictions, venous backup.
   c. Background: uneven pigmentation, hemorrhages, cotton-wool areas, exudates, retinal edema, detached retina.
   d. Macula: uneven pigmentation, hemorrhage, exudates, edema.

4. Discuss the significance of opacities; describe the technique for eliciting the red reflex and locating the depth of corneal and lens opacities.

5. Describe the proper technique for handling the ophthalmoscope and give rationales for
   a. room lighting.
   b. choice of lens (diopters) and diaphragm (light beam) settings.
   c. preparation of the client.

6. Describe the procedure for assessment of intraocular pressure by light palpation; discuss implications of abnormal pressures.

LEARNING ACTIVITIES

The Learning Activities contain the information necessary for meeting the Cognitive Objectives. Select one and work with it until you have mastered the material. Use the

Cognitive Objectives as a study guide. A Self-Test is provided so that you can check how much you know. If you have difficulty with the Self-Test, please review the material in this unit.

Reading Activities

a) Bates: *A Guide to Physical Examination*. Read p. 19 for anatomy and physiology, pp. 35–38 for examination techniques, and pp. 53 and 57–61 for tables of common abnormal findings. Supplement with reading about assessment of intraocular pressure by palpation.

b) DeGowin and DeGowin: *Bedside Diagnostic Examination*. Read pp. 102–103 for palpation of intraocular pressure, pp. 103–116 for ophthalmoscopic examination, pp. 96–97 for corneal opacities and pp. 101–102 for opacities of the lens. This activity is geared to the experienced practitioner.

c) Delp and Manning: *Major's Physical Diagnosis*, Chapter 7, "The Eyes." This reading offers a detailed description of opacities. Explanation of the funduscopic examination is brief and assumes prior knowledge of the procedure and normal findings. Extensive supplementation is required to meet the objectives.

d) Gillies and Alyn: *Patient Assessment and Management by the Nurse Practitioner*, "Examination of the Head and Neck," pp. 46–51. This reading presents a concise overview of examination of the fundus. Opacities and intraocular pressure are not discussed. The beginning practitioner may wish to obtain specific information about handling the ophthalmoscope before reading this chapter. Additional reading is suggested for greater understanding.

e) Judge and Zuidema: *Methods of Clinical Examination: A Physiologic Approach*, Chapter 6, "The Eye," pp. 68–72, 76–79. This section briefly discusses technique and normal findings. It is geared to the practitioner who wishes more information about pathological features.

f) Prior and Silberstein: *Physical Diagnosis*, Chapter 6, "Eyes," pp. 96–127. In this comprehensive coverage of the ophthalmoscopic examination procedures and normal and abnormal findings are clearly described and diagrammed.

g) Sana and Judge: *Physical Appraisal Methods in Nursing Practice*, Chapter 6, "The Eye," pp. 61, 68–72, 76–79. Techniques for locating opacities and performing examination of the fundus are brief and better suited to the experienced practitioner. Abnormal findings are well described.

h) Sherman and Fields: *Guide to Patient Evaluation*, "The Eyes," pp. 78–79, 84–90. This brief but systematic examination of the disc, vessels and macula offers a good introduction for the student beginning to use the ophthalmoscope. The reader will need to supplement learning in all areas.

Audiovisual Activities

a) "Ophthalmoscopy: Basic Self-Instruction," distributed by the National Audiovisual Center. This comprehensive program consists of slides, audiocassettes, a study guide and mannequins. Since this is a lengthy unit, the student should not try to complete it in one session. The following approach is suggested.

1. Complete the slide-tape sets entitled "Overview," "Introduction," "Disc," "Vessels," "General Background" and "Summary" (study time, 2½ hr).

2. Complete "Using the Ophthalmoscope," which covers handling the instrument, location of opacities and mannequin practice. Follow the study guide, pp. 29–42 (study time, 1½ to 2 hr).

3. When you feel confident with the mannequin, practice on a live subject; follow the study guide, pp. 46–48.

Supplemental Activities

The following materials are suggested to strengthen your learning.
a) "Cataracts," Clinical Symposium Reprints, CIBA Pharmaceutical Co.
b) "Diseases of the Eye," Clinical Symposium Reprints, CIBA Pharmaceutical Co.

SELF-TEST

This Self-Test is for you. Use it to check how well you have learned the material presented in this unit. The answers follow the test.

1. The following diagram represents the fundus of the ___*rt*___ eye.

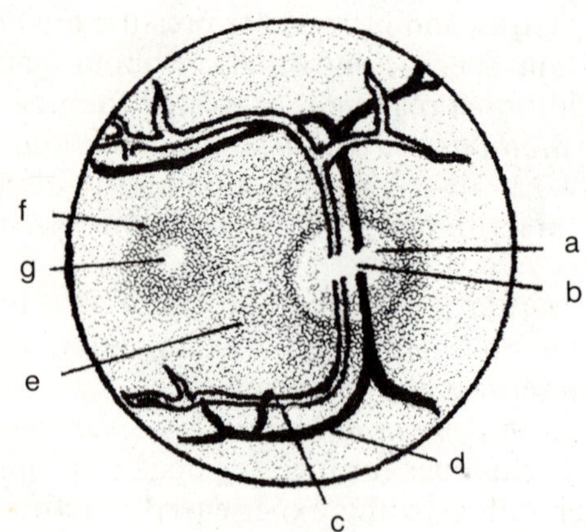

2. In the preceding diagram, name the lettered structures.

   a) *disc*

   b) *cup*

   c) *artery*

   d) *vein*

   e) *background*

   f) *macula*

   g) *fovea*

3. In a through d, identify features of the optic disc.

   a) The shape is normally ___*oval*___ with ___*distinct*___ margins.

   b) The cup:disc ratio should be ___*1:2*___ .

   c) The color is ___*darker pink*___ than the general background.

   d) Scleral and pigmented crescents outlining the optic disc are considered (normal/ abnormal).

4. In a through e, identify features of the retinal vessels.
   a) The vessels narrow in caliber as they reach the (perimeter/disc).

   b) The AV ratio is normally _2 : 3_ .
   c) The blood column should be (regular/irregular).

   d) AV crossings which interrupt blood flow can be identified by _venous engorgement_
   e) Light is reflected by the (veins/arteries).

5. In a through d, identify features of the general background.

   a) Pigmentation corresponds with _individual pigmentation_

   b) Visualization of the choroidal vascular pattern is most often seen in _blondes_ .

   c) A normal finding in elderly clients is _drusen_ .

   d) Fluffy white patches caused by vascular occlusion are called _cotton wool_ .

6. The macula
   1. is located to the temporal side of the fundus.
   2. appears to be an area of great vascularity.
   3. is examined for pigmentation and integrity.
   4. is relatively insensitive to light.
   5. frequently contains microaneurysms, or flame-shaped hemorrhages.
   a) 1, 2 and 5 are correct.
   b) 1 and 3 are correct.
   c) 2, 3 and 5 are correct.
   d) 2 and 4 are correct.
   e) all of the above are correct.

7. A dark shadow that interrupts the red reflex (fundus glow) is usually
   a) a sign of glaucoma.
   b) a sign of hemorrhage in the retina.
   c) an opacity.
   d) a normal finding.

Match the terms in 8 through 10 with the appropriate description.

8. ___C___ Corneal opacity

9. ___B___ Anterior lens opacity

10. ___A___ Posterior lens or vitreous opacity

a) Opacity appears to move in the same direction as the examiner.
b) Opacity does not appear to move.
c) Opacity can be seen with direct illumination.

11. The lens settings on the ophthalmoscope are called diopters.
   1. Negative diopters (red numbers) have a greater focal length than positive diopters.
   2. Opacities are usually seen with the positive diopters.
   3. The retina is usually best visualized with the negative diopters.

a) 1 only is correct.
b) 2 only is correct.
c) 3 only is correct.
d) 1 and 2 are correct.
e) all of the above are correct.

12. To examine the fundus, you should approach the client from a position about _15°___________ from his straight line of view.

13. If you noted increased intraocular pressure or a cup:disc ratio greater than 1:2, you would suspect that the client might have _glaucoma_.

14. Findings associated with hypertension include
   1. cotton-wool areas.
   2. focal or generalized narrowing of the arterioles.
   3. thickened arterioles with broad light reflexes (copper wiring).
   4. AV crossings which show interference with blood flow.
a) 2 only is correct.
b) 1 and 2 are correct.
c) 4 only is correct.
d) 3 and 4 are correct.
e) all of the above are correct.

15. _Papilledema_____ is the result of venous stasis with engorgement and swelling of the optic disc.

SELF-TEST KEY

1. Right eye.   In each eye, the disc is located on the nasal side of the fundus.

2. (a) disc
   (b) cup
   (c) retinal artery
   (d) retinal vein
   (e) general background
   (f) macula
   (g) fovea

3. (a) The shape of the optic disc is normally oval or round with fairly distinct margins.
   (b) less than 1:2.
   (c) darker pink
   (d) normal.

4. (a) perimeter.
   (b) 2:3 or 4:5.
   (c) regular.
   (d) venous engorgement.
   (e) arteries.   Light is reflected as a white stripe along the vessel.

5. (a) individual skin pigmentation.
   (b) persons with blond hair.

    (c) drusen (tiny, round, yellowish spots).
    (d) cotton-wool areas.

6. (b) The macula is on the temporal side of the fundus and is examined for pigmentation and integrity. The normal macular area appears to have few blood vessels. Shining a light on the tiny sensitive center of the macula, the fovea, is very painful, and this is a good reason for examining this area last. Tiny red dots frequently located in the macular area represent microaneurysms. They are characteristic of diabetic retinal damage. Flame-shaped (linear) hemorrhages are superficial changes associated with severe hypertension.

7. (c) Dark shadows which interrupt the red reflex are abnormal and indicate opacities of the cornea, lens or deeper structures. They are not specific for glaucoma or retinal hemorrhage.

8. (c) See answer to 10.

9. (b) See answer to 10.

10. (a) Corneal opacities appear as white spots when a light is shone directly on the cornea. Opacities in the lens or deeper appear as dark shadows which interrupt the red reflex when the ophthalmoscope light is shone on the pupil from a distance of 4 to 6 inches. The depth of an opacity is estimated by manipulating the ophthalmoscope and observing the apparent movement of the opacity. Corneal opacities seem to move in a direction opposite to the examiner's direction of movement. Anterior lens opacities are stationary. Opacities in the posterior lens or deeper in the vitreous humor appear to move in the same direction as the examiner.

11. (e) Negative diopters are minifiers and have a greater focal length which allows the examiner to see the retina of the eye. The positive diopters are magnifiers and are used to see areas closer to the anterior portion of the eye.

12. To examine the fundus, the examiner should approach the client from an angle of 15° away from his line of vision. Opacities are best examined by approaching the client directly in the client's line of view.

13. glaucoma.

14. (b) Cotton-wool areas and arteriolar narrowing are associated with retinal changes in hypertension. Copper wiring and AV crossings are associated with arteriosclerosis.

15. Papilledema, or "choked disc," is caused by increased intracranial pressure. Swelling of the optic nerve obstructs flow of blood from the eye along the central retinal vein. Since the optic nerve is not functionally impaired, there is rarely impairment of vision.

CLINICAL COMPONENT

    The Clinical Component for Units 7 through 11 is presented in Unit 12 (Head and Neck: Clinical Component, p. 217). Preview the Clinical Objectives in that unit and the Performance Guide cards for Unit 12 in Appendix II. Facilitate your learning by practicing these skills before proceeding to the next unit.

PRE-TEST

UNIT 9

1. The function(s) of the ear is (are)
   a) hearing.
   b) balance.
   c) both a and b.

2. The Weber test is normal when the sound
   a) lateralizes to one ear.
   b) is heard equally well in both ears.

3. In the Rinne test air conduction normally lasts______________________bone conduction.
   a) longer than
   b) shorter than
   c) the same length of time as

4. The light reflex in the left ear is cone-shaped and is in the ___5___ o'clock position.
   a) 5
   b) 7
   c) 3
   d) 11
   e) none of the above.

5. When the eustachian tube is blocked, the eardrum will
   a) bulge.
   b) retract.
   c) remain unaltered.

6. A bluish tympanic membrane indicates
   a) pus behind the drum.
   b) blood in the middle ear.
   c) air bubbles behind the drum.
   d) otitis media.

7. The ear bone most often visualized on inspection of the normal ear is the
   a) incus.
   b) stapes.
   c) malleus.

8. The client who has a serous discharge from an ear should alert the examiner to
   1. obtain a culture.
   2. test drainage for glucose.
   3. irrigate the ear with tepid normal saline.
   4. suspect a skull fracture and arrange an immediate referral.
   a) 1 only is correct.
   b) 1 and 3 are correct.
   c) 2 and 4 are correct.

    d) 1, 2 and 4 are correct.
    e) all of the above are correct.

9. Conductive hearing can be impaired by
    1. otosclerosis.
    2. perforation of the eardrum.
    3. obstruction of the auditory canal.
    a) 2 only is correct.
    b) 1 and 3 are correct.
    c) 2 and 3 are correct.
    d) all of the above are correct.

10. Landmarks of the tympanic membrane include the
    1. semicircular canal.
    2. helix.
    3. cochlea.
    4. malleus.
    a) 1 and 3 are correct.
    b) 4 only is correct.
    c) 1 and 2 are correct.
    d) 3 only is correct.

11. For proper visualization of the auditory canal in adults, the ear must be pulled
    a) up and back.
    b) straight back.
    c) down and back.
    d) forward and up.

12. A bulging, bright red tympanic membrane indicates
    a) skull fracture.
    b) acute otitis media.
    c) swimmer's ear.
    d) obstruction of the eustachian tube.

13. The entire outer ear is called the
    a) helix.
    b) lobe.
    c) pinna.
    d) tragus.

14. With the Weber test, better hearing on the right side indicates
    1. neurosensory loss on the left.
    2. neurosensory loss on the right.
    3. conductive loss on the left.
    4. conductive loss on the right.
    a) 1 only is correct.
    b) 1 and 4 are correct.
    c) 2 and 3 are correct.
    d) 3 only is correct.

15. Neurosensory hearing depends on the function of
    a) the inner ear.
    b) the VIII cranial nerve (acoustic nerve).

c) the brain.
d) all of the above.

16. Ear pain is termed
   a) otorrhea.
   b) tinnitus.
   c) otalgia.
   d) otitis media.

17. Structures of the inner ear include the
   1. umbo.
   2. cochlea.
   3. stapes.
   4. tympanic membrane.
   a) 2 and 3 are correct.
   b) 2, 3 and 4 are correct.
   c) 2 only is correct.
   d) all of the above are correct.

Identify the following structures in the accompanying illustration.

18. ___D___ Pars tensa

19. ___C___ Anulus

20. ___B___ Malleus

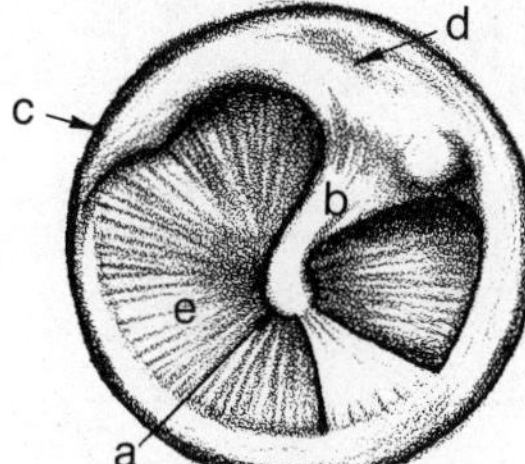

Number 9

Examination of the Ears

RATIONALE

This self-instructional unit is designed to help you learn inspection of the ear. This unit concentrates on tests for hearing and balance and the assessment of the external and middle ear. After completing this unit, you will be able to evaluate a client's gross hearing and balance, assess the external and middle ear and describe any abnormalities present.

GLOSSARY OF TERMS

Review the following terms before and after completing this unit. You should be able to define or describe them readily.

Anulus _ring of tissue around an opening_

Cerumen _ear wax_

Cochlea _portion of temporal bone housing membranous & osseous labyrinth_

Eustachian tube _auditory tube_

Helix _rounded convex margin of pinna of ear_

Incus _middle bone of middle ear_

Malleus _"hammer"_

Mastoid _breast shaped bone behind the ear_

Otalgia _earache_

Otitis externa _external inflammation of the ear_

Otitis media _middle ear infection_

Otorrhea _discharge from external auditory meatus_

Pars flaccida _flaccid part of tympanic membrane_

Pinna _visible part of ear_

Stapes *stirrup*

Tinnitus *ringing in the ear*

Tympanic membrane *eardrum*

Umbo *projection in center of eardrum*

Vertigo *dizziness*

COGNITIVE OBJECTIVES

At the end of this unit you will demonstrate knowledge of inspection and palpation of the external ear and auditory acuity by your ability to:

1. Identify the functions of the ear.

2. Label the parts of the external, middle and inner ear and associated structures on a diagram.

3. Discuss mechanisms of conductive (air conduction) and sensorineural (bone conduction) hearing; describe the Weber and Rinne tests and identify the normal and abnormal findings for each.

4. Systematically list and describe the landmarks seen on inspection of the normal tympanic membrane: umbo, malleus, light reflex, pars tensa, pars flaccida, anulus.

5. Describe manipulation of pinna and canal for otoscopic examination, including the method and precautions; discuss the procedure for evaluating eustachian tube patency.

6. Describe symptoms and examination findings which are associated with infection, trauma and blocked eustachian tube.

LEARNING ACTIVITIES

The Learning Activities contain the information necessary for meeting the Cognitive Objectives. Select one and proceed to work with it until you have mastered the material. Use the Cognitive Objectives as a study guide. A Self-Test is provided so that you can check how much you know. If you have difficulty with the Self-Test, please review the material in this unit.

Reading Activities

a) Bates: *A Guide to Physical Examination*, Chapter 4 (pp. 23–24, 39–40, 62–64) discusses the anatomy of the ear, hearing tests, inspection of the external ear and tympanic membrane and abnormal findings. The text contains many drawings which facilitate understanding.

b) DeGowin and DeGowin: *Bedside Diagnostic Examination* (pp. 173–188) presents extensive coverage of all aspects of ear examination with emphasis on diagnosis of abnormalities.

c) Delp and Manning: *Major's Physical Diagnosis*, Chapter 5, "General Principles of the Ear, Nose and Throat Examination." This reading presents a brief overview of the principles of external and otoscopic ear examination; heavy supplementation is required.

d) Gillies and Alyn: *Patient Assessment and Management by the Nurse Practitioner*, "Examination of the Head and Neck," pp. 51–53. This section contains a cursory description of examination of the canal and tympanic membrane. The Weber and Rinne tests are discussed. Supplement your reading in all areas to meet the objectives.

e) Judge and Zuidema: *Methods of Clinical Examination: A Physiologic Approach*, Chapter 8, "Ears, Nose and Throat," pp. 91, 94–95, 100–101, 102–103. This chapter contains an overview of the otoscopic examination procedures and findings. You will need to supplement your reading in all areas.

f) Prior and Silberstein: *Physical Diagnosis*, Chapter 8, "Ears, Nose and Throat," pp. 132–145. Assessment of the landmarks of the eardrum and testing of hearing acuity are well covered. Supplement your reading to include structure of the external ear and examination findings.

g) Sana and Judge: *Physical Appraisal Methods in Nursing Practice*, Chapter 8, "Physical Appraisal of the Ear and Hearing," pp. 121–130. This chapter offers a comprehensive assessment of procedures and findings for hearing acuity and external and otoscopic examinations; a glossary is also included. The beginning student may require additional explanation of techniques.

h) Sherman and Fields: *Guide to Physical Evaluation*, Chapter 10, "The Ear, Nose, Mouth and Pharynx," pp. 91–96. Topographical anatomy, the Weber test and examination findings are clearly presented. You will need to supplement your learning by reading about functions of the ear, the Rinne test, procedures for checking eustachian tube patency and common pathological findings.

i) Mechner, Francis: "Examination of the Ear," *AJN*, Vol. 75, No. 3, pp. 1–24, March 1975. This programmed instruction presents comprehensive coverage of anatomy, examination techniques and common abnormalities. The Weber and Rinne tests are explained in detail.

Audiovisual Activities

a) Blue-Hill Educational Systems, Inc.: "Ears – Part V" (video tape). This program presents a comprehensive lecture covering evaluation of hearing, different types of hearing loss, inspection of the auditory canal and tympanic membrane, abnormal findings and evaluation of the vestibular system. The techniques of the Weber and Rinne tests are demonstrated.

b) Concept Media: "The Ear," film strip.

Supplemental Activities

The following materials are suggested to strengthen your learning.

a) Abbott Laboratory: *Some Pathological Conditions of the Eye, Ear and Throat* (an atlas) contains excellent color photographs.

b) CIBA Pharmaceutical Co.: "Otologic Diagnosis and Treatment of Deafness," Clinical Symposium Reprints.

c) Fowkes and Hunn: *Clinical Assessment for the Nurse Practitioner*, pp. 44–48, contains a good review of anatomy and a brief overview of examination techniques and pathophysiology.

SELF-TEST

This Self-Test is for you. Use it to check how well you have learned the material presented in the unit. The answers follow the test.

1. Functions of the ear are _____*hearing*_____ and _____*balance*_____ .

2. Identify the structures lettered in the accompanying diagram.

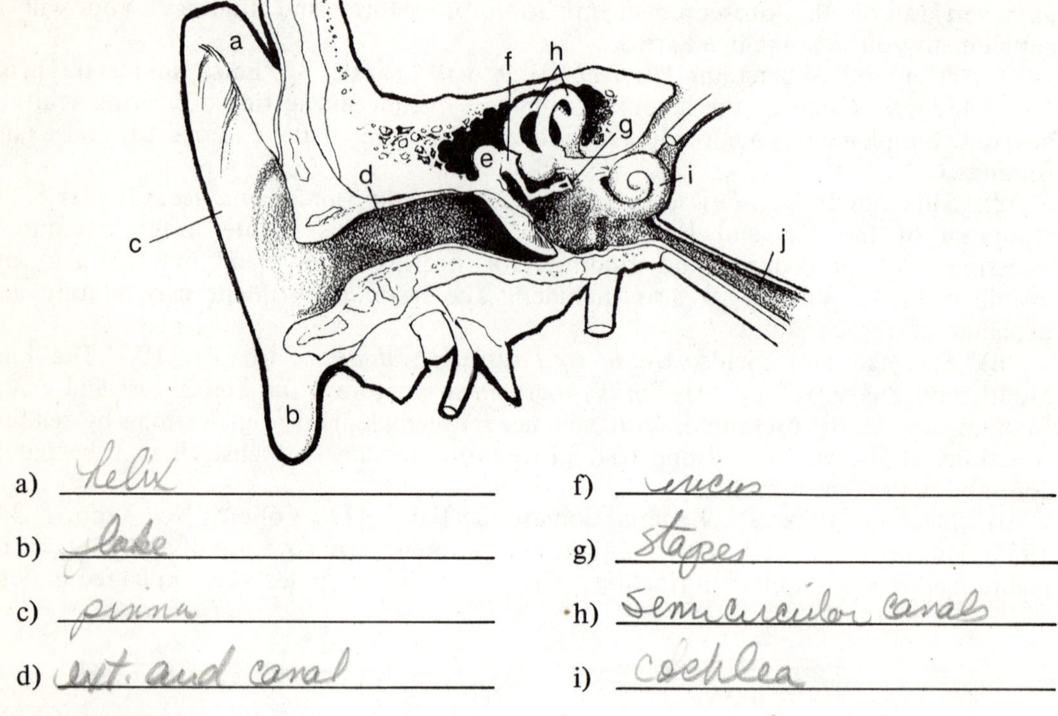

a) _____*helix*_____

b) _____*lobe*_____

c) _____*pinna*_____

d) _____*ext. aud canal*_____

e) _____*malleus*_____

f) _____*incus*_____

g) _____*stapes*_____

h) _____*semicircular canals*_____

i) _____*cochlea*_____

j) _____*eustachian tube*_____

3. Identify the landmarks of the eardrum labeled in the following drawing.

a) __*2*__ malleus

b) __*4*__ umbo

c) __*3*__ pars flaccida

d) __*6*__ anulus

e) __*5*__ pars tensa

f) _____ light reflex

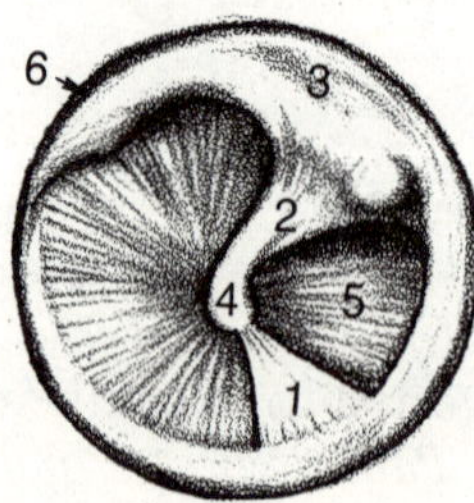

4. Rank in order the structures along the pathway for *air-conducted* sound vibrations.

    a) __3__ tympanic membrane

    b) __1__ external ear

    c) __5__ incus

    d) __7__ oval window

    e) __8__ cochlea

    f) __4__ malleus

    g) __2__ auditory canal

    h) __6__ stapes

    i) __9__ VIII cranial nerve

5. Sensorineural hearing is the function of _Organ of Corti_ and _VIII Cranial nerve_

6. Bone conduction normally takes twice as long as air conduction.
    a) True
    b) False

7. In the Weber test, lateralization of sound to the left ear indicates a
        1. conduction loss in the left ear.
        2. conduction loss in the right ear.
        3. sensorineural loss in the left ear.
        4. sensorineural loss in the right ear.
        5. normal variant.
    a) 1 and 3 are correct.
    b) 1 and 4 are correct.
    c) 2 and 3 are correct.
    d) 2 and 4 are correct.
    e) 5 only is correct.

8. Conductive loss may be due to _failure of transmission of vibration_

9. The light reflex in the right ear
    a) is cone-shaped at the 7 o'clock position.
    b) is located at the 5 o'clock position.
    c) may be absent as a normal variant.
    d) is described correctly in a and c.
    e) is described correctly in b and c.

10. The most prominent ear bone that is visualized in the normal ear is the
    a) incus.
    b) stapes.
    c) malleus.
    d) mastoid.

11. Selection of the appropriate size of speculum for the otoscope is based on using
    a) the smallest one available.
    b) one which is most comfortable for the patient.
    c) whatever is available and clean.
    d) the largest one which fits comfortably.
    e) the correct size in relation to the age of the client.

12. In adults manipulation of the pinna for insertion of the otoscope requires that the examiner pull the ear
    a) down and back.
    b) up, out and back.
    c) straight out and back.
    d) down and forward.

13. Describe how you would check for patency of the eustachian tube.

14. Blockage of the eustachian tube
    a) causes retraction of the drum.
    b) creates a negative pressure in the middle ear.
    c) causes initial bulging of the drum.
    d) produces the effects in both a and b.
    e) produces the effects in both b and c.

15. When a client presents with a bloody or serous drainage from the ear, the examiner

    must first rule out _skull fracture_ as the cause.

Match the following columns:

16. __C__ Air bubbles behind the drum
17. __B__ Blue drum
18. __D__ Red, bulging drum
19. __C__ Amber drum
20. __E__ Dark spots on the drum
21. __A__ Reddened, tender canal

    a) Otitis externa
    b) Hemorrhagic otitis media
    c) Serous otitis media
    d) Acute purulent otitis media
    e) Perforations

Match the following columns:

22. __E__ Drainage from the ear
23. __C__ Ear pain
24. __A__ Inflammation of the ear

    a) Otitis
    b) Vertigo
    c) Otalgia
    d) Tinnitus
    e) Otorrhea

25. ___D___ "Ringing" in the ears

26. ___B___ Feeling of spinning or dizziness

SELF-TEST KEY

1. The functions of the ear are hearing and balance.

2. (a) helix
   (b) lobe
   (c) pinna
   (d) external auditory canal
   (e) malleus
   (f) incus
   (g) stapes
   (h) semicircular canals
   (i) cochlea
   (j) eustachian tube

3. (a) 2
   (b) 4
   (c) 3
   (d) 6
   (e) 5
   (f) 1

4. 1, external ear; 2, auditory canal; 3, tympanic membrane; 4, malleus; 5, incus; 6, stapes; 7, oval window; 8, cochlea; 9, VIII cranial nerve.

5. Sensorineural hearing is the function of the organ of Corti and the VIII cranial nerve. The organ of Corti in the cochlea of the inner ear receives sound vibrations transmitted by bone and sends them to the brain via the cochlear branch of the VIII cranial (acoustic) nerve.

6. (b) False. Air conduction of sound normally takes twice as long as bone conduction of sound. This is the rationale for a normal Rinne test.

7. (b) In a normal Weber test, the sound from the tuning fork placed on the midline of the head does not lateralize. Since the sound is perceived by bone conduction (sensorineural), lateralization to one side may indicate a sensorineural loss in the opposite ear (4). However, since loss of air conduction (conductive) in one ear allows the sensory receptors to be more sensitive in that ear, a conductive loss is possible in the ear to which the sound lateralizes (1).

8. Conductive loss occurs with failure of transmission of sound vibrations to the sensory apparatus in the inner ear. This can be caused by blockage of the external ear, disorders of the drum or middle ear disease. (*Note*: since hearing ultimately depends on relay of information to the brain, conductive hearing is said to have two components — air conduction and bone conduction. However, a *pure conductive loss* only involves the external or middle ear, as discussed above.)

9. (b) The light reflex in the right ear is cone-shaped and points to the 5 o'clock position.

10. (c) The manubrium, or handle of the malleus, is the most prominent ear bone visualized during examination. With retraction of the eardrum, the other bones may be identified.

11. (d) The determining factor is not the age of the client but the size of the ear canal. Too small a speculum prevents adequate examination and necessitates manipulation within the ear, usually causing great discomfort! By using the largest speculum *which fits comfortably*, the examiner obtains the best visibility and with reasonable care is not likely to hurt the client. A sterile speculum is rarely necessary, but there is no excuse for using dirty instruments.

12. (b) In infants, the pinna is pulled down to straighten the canal.

13. If the eustachian tube is blocked, air cannot enter the middle ear from the nasopharynx. Instruct the client to blow forcibly against closed nose and mouth while observing for movement of the tympanic membrane. Movement indicates patency of the tube.

14. (d) When the eustachian tube is blocked, the air in the middle ear is absorbed into the surrounding tissue, creating a negative pressure and retracting the drums. Bulging of the drum occurs when the middle ear fills with fluid, blood or purulent material.

15. Serous or bloody ear drainage frequently results from skull fracture. The presence of glucose in a serous drainage indicates that it is cerebrospinal fluid. All drainage from the ears should be cultured. If a skull fracture is suspected, immediate referral is recommended.

16. (c)

17. (b)

18. (d)

19. (c)

20. (e)

21. (a)

22. (e)

23. (c)

24. (a)

25. (d)

26. (b)

CLINICAL COMPONENT

The Clinical Component for Units 7 through 11 is presented in Unit 12, Head and Neck: Clinical Component. Preview the Clinical Objectives in that unit and the Performance Guide cards for Unit 12 in Appendix II. Facilitate your learning by practicing these skills before proceeding to the next unit.

PRE-TEST

UNIT 10

Choose the *one* most correct answer.

1. A pustule in the nasal vestibule is called a
   a) polyp.
   b) furuncle.
   c) chancre.
   d) canker sore.

2. Sinus tenderness is tested by pressing upward against the frontal and maxillary areas.
   a) True
   b) False

3. Nasal mucosa which is swollen, pale and boggy is associated with
   a) the common cold.
   b) an allergic response.
   c) measles.
   d) none of the above.

4. Herpes simplex causes
   a) a small cluster of blisters on or near the lips which break and crust.
   b) fissuring and crusting primarily of the lower lip.
   c) a buttonlike crusted chancre on or near the mouth.
   d) fissuring and crusting at the angles of the mouth.

5. Mrs. Clark brings her 6-year-old son into the emergency room for treatment. His symptoms are malaise, fever, myalgia, cough and photophobia. Inspection reveals white granular spots on the buccal mucosa opposite the upper molars. You suspect
   a) mumps.
   b) acute rhinitis.
   c) rubeola.
   d) scarlet fever.

6. The nasal septum
   a) is inspected for bleeding and perforation.
   b) is nontender.
   c) may interfere with breathing if it is deviated.
   d) is correctly described in a and c.
   e) is correctly described in all of the above.

7. The ducts from the parotid glands are located
   a) at the base of the tongue.
   b) in the buccal mucosa opposite the upper second molar.
   c) between the middle and superior turbinates.

8. A thin, white coating on the tongue is
   a) always abnormal.

    b) a sign of vitamin C deficiency.
    c) normal for most people.
    d) leukoplakia.

9. Paralysis of the XII cranial (hypoglossal) nerve results in
    a) deviation of the uvula to the affected side.
    b) deviation of the tongue to the affected side.
    c) loss of sense of taste on the anterior 2/3 of the tongue.
    d) deviation of the tongue to the unaffected side.

10. Thickened white plaques on the tongue or mucosa which may be premalignant are called
    a) Koplik spots.
    b) crypts.
    c) thrush.
    d) leukoplakia.

11. Tonsils are inspected for
        1. presence.
        2. size.
        3. crypts.
        4. exudates.
    a) 3 and 4 are correct.
    b) 1 and 2 are correct.
    c) 2, 3 and 4 are correct.
    d) all of the above are correct.

12. Suspicious lesions in or about the mouth should always be examined with a gloved hand.
    a) True
    b) False

13. Nasal polyps are generally associated with
    a) the common cold.
    b) infection of the mastoid sinus.
    c) tonsillitis.
    d) chronic allergies.

14. Vitamin B_{12} deficiency can be detected by observing
    a) a geographic tongue.
    b) a black hairy tongue.
    c) a smooth, beefy red tongue.
    d) purplish swellings under the tongue.

15. Teeth which are abnormally small, widely spaced and notched on the biting surfaces are a sign of
    a) dental caries.
    b) congenital syphilis.
    c) vitamin or calcium deficiency.

16. Fissures or cracking at the angles of the mouth is called
    a) herpes simplex.
    b) syphilitic chancre.

    c) cheilosis.
    d) cheilitis.

17. Gingivitis is characterized by
    a) redness and swelling of the margins of the gums.
    b) brownish melanin pigmentation of the gums.
    c) thick white patches on the mucous membranes.
    d) hypertrophy of the tongue.

18. White plaques in the mouth resembling milk curds
    a) are known as Koplik spots.
    b) are canker sores.
    c) are associated with mononucleosis.
    d) indicate a yeast infection.

19. With paralysis of the X cranial (vagus) nerve, the uvula deviates to ______________ side when the patient says "ah."
    a) the involved
    b) the uninvolved
    c) neither

20. Inflammation of the back of the throat is called
    a) laryngitis.
    b) pyorrhea.
    c) pharyngitis.
    d) epiglottitis.

Number 10

The Examination of the Nose, Mouth and Pharynx

RATIONALE

The purpose of this self-instructional unit is to help you learn inspection and palpation of the nose, mouth and pharynx. At the end of the unit, you will be able to evaluate these structures for normality and describe several common abnormalities.

GLOSSARY OF TERMS

Review the following terms before and after completing this unit. You should be able to define or describe them readily.

Adenoids ____

Aphthous ulcers (canker sores) ____

Buccal ____

Caries ____

Crypts ____

Chancre ____

Cheilitis ____

Cheilosis (angular stomatitis) ____

Fissure ____

Fordyce spots ____

Furuncle ____

Gingivitis ____

Herpes simplex ____

Hutchinson's teeth ____

Koplik's spots ____

Leukoplakia ____

Moniliasis ____

Papillae ____

Parotid glands ____

Periodontitis ____

Pharyngitis ____

Plaque ____

Polyp ____

Pyorrhea ____

Rhinitis ____

Thrush ____

Turbinate ____

Uvula ____

COGNITIVE OBJECTIVES

At the end of this unit you will demonstrate inspection and palpation of the nose, mouth and pharynx by your ability to:

1. Systematically list and describe normal examination findings for the external and internal structures of the
   a. nose: mucosa, turbinates, meatuses, septum, maxillary sinuses.
   b. mouth: lips, mucosa, gums, teeth, salivary glands, tongue, hard palate.
   c. pharynx: soft palate, pillars, uvula, posterior pharynx.

2. Discuss signs and symptoms which indicate dysfunction.

3. Discuss the procedures for inspection of the internal nose and palpation of the sinuses.

4. Describe methods for testing neurological innervation of nose, mouth and pharynx.

LEARNING ACTIVITIES

The Learning Activities contain information necessary for meeting the Cognitive Objectives. Select one and proceed to work with it until you have mastered the material. Use the Cognitive Objectives as a study guide. A Self-Test is provided so you can check how much you know. If you have difficulty with the Self-Test, please review the material in this unit.

Reading Activities

a) Bates: *A Guide to Physical Examination*. Read pp. 25–27 for a review of anatomy and physiology, pp. 41–44 for examination techniques and pp. 65–71 for a discussion of abnormal findings. Also read pp. 270–272 and 274–275 for a discussion of the neurological innervation of the nose and mouth. Numerous illustrations are presented throughout.

b) DeGowin and DeGowin: *Bedside Diagnostic Examination*, Chapter 5, "The Head and Neck," pp. 118–172. In-depth coverage of anatomy and physiology, techniques and procedures, and examination findings is presented. Emphasis is placed on differential diagnosis. This is an excellent reference for the experienced practitioner.

c) Delp and Manning: *Major's Physical Diagnosis*, Chapter 4, "Examination of the Head and Neck," presents an overview of examination findings. Photographs of abnormalities are excellent. You will need to supplement your learning extensively to meet the objectives.

d) Gillies and Alyn: *Patient Assessment and Management by the Nurse Practitioner*, pp. 53–58. Knowledge of anatomy and examination procedures is assumed. Normal and common abnormal findings are discussed in detail.

e) Judge and Zuidema: *Methods of Clinical Examination: A Physiologic Approach*, Chapter 7, "Mouth and Jaws," pp. 81–88 and Chapter 8, "Ears, Nose and Throat," pp. 91–93, 97–98, 100–102. These chapters offer a comprehensive discussion of the procedures, normal and abnormal findings. A glossary of pertinent terms and anatomical diagrams aid understanding.

f) Prior and Silberstein: *Physical Diagnosis*, Chapter 8, "Ears, Nose and Throat," pp. 128–132, 145–152, 161–168. This chapter provides comprehensive coverage of all aspects of examination of the nose, mouth and pharynx.

g) Sana and Judge: *Physical Appraisal Methods in Nursing Practice* does not include a specific chapter on examination of the nose, mouth and pharynx.

h) Sherman and Fields: *Guide to Patient Evaluation*, Chapter 10, "The Ear, Nose, Mouth and Pharynx," pp. 96–100. This chapter discusses procedures, techniques and examination findings in a clear, concise manner. The focus is on normal findings. Supplemental reading about abnormal findings is advised.

Audiovisual Activities

a) Blue-Hill Educational Systems, Inc.: "Nose – Part 6" and "Mouth and Throat – Part 7" (video tape). This program presents a comprehensive approach to inspection and palpation. Anatomical locations and physiological functioning of the structures of the nose, mouth and pharynx are discussed. Normal findings of inspection and palpation are stressed and briefly contrasted with common abnormal states. A demonstration of a systematic evaluation is given, including the proper use of the otoscope with nasal attachment.

Supplemental Activities

The following materials are suggested to strengthen your learning.

a) Mechner, Francis: "Patient Assessment: Examination of the Head and Neck." *AJN*, Vol. 75, No. 5, May 1975 (programmed instruction).

b) CIBA Pharmaceutical Co.: "White Lesions of the Mouth," Clinical Symposium Reprints.

c) CIBA Pharmaceutical Co.: "Diseases and Surgery of the Nose," Clinical Symposium Reprints.

SELF-TEST

This Self-Test is for you. Use it to check how well you have learned the material presented in the unit. The answers follow the test.

1. When inspecting the internal nares the examiner should remember
    a) the nasal septum is very sensitive.
    b) the inferior, middle and superior turbinates should all be readily visible.
    c) features in both a and b.
    d) none of the above.

2. The paranasal sinuses drain into
    a) the inferior meatus.
    b) the middle turbinate.
    c) the middle meatus.
    d) none of the above structures.

3. Polyps in the nose are usually associated with
    a) allergic rhinitis.
    b) acute rhinitis.
    c) mastoiditis.

4. Fissures or cracking at the angles of the mouth is called
    a) herpes simplex.
    b) syphilitic chancre.
    c) cheilosis.
    d) none of the above.

5. Examination of the mouth should be done with dentures in place.
    a) True
    b) False

6. White plaques in the mouth resembling milk curds
    a) are canker sores.
    b) are known as Fordyce spots.
    c) indicate a yeast infection.

7. Gingivitis is characterized by
    a) redness and swelling of the margins of the gums.
    b) brownish melanin pigmentation of the gums.
    c) purulent inflammation of the gums and loosened teeth.

8. The teeth are assessed for
    a) color, placement and caries.
    b) presence, shape, position, looseness and caries.
    c) absence, position and color.
    d) symmetry, color and lesions.

9. Teeth which are abnormally notched on the biting surfaces are a sign of
    a) dental caries.
    b) congenital syphilis.
    c) vitamin or calcium deficiency.
    d) all of the above.

10. A thin, white coating on the tongue is
  a) always abnormal.
  b) a sign of vitamin C deficiency.
  c) normal for most people.
  d) leukoplakia.

11. A smooth, red tongue suggests
  a) fungal disease.
  b) vitamin B_{12} deficiency.
  c) dehydration.

12. With paralysis of the X cranial (vagus) nerve, the uvula
  a) deviates to the involved side.
  b) deviates to the uninvolved side.
  c) does not deviate but rises symmetrically.

SELF-TEST KEY

1. (a) Care must be taken to avoid touching the nasal septum with the speculum. Generally, the superior turbinate is not visualized in routine examination but requires use of a nasopharyngeal mirror.

2. (c) The paranasal sinuses drain into the middle meatus. The nasolacrimal ducts drain into the inferior meatus. The turbinates are bony shelves which project into the nasal cavity.

3. (a) Soft, mobile, pale gray polyps are found frequently in the middle meatus of patients with allergic rhinitis. Symptoms of acute rhinitis include a red and swollen nasal mucosa. Mastoiditis is an infection of the bony mastoid air cells in the temporal bone.

4. (c) Cheilosis is a fissuring or cracking of the skin at the corners of the mouth. It is frequently caused by excess moisture on the skin from malocclusion, ill-fitting dentures, poor hygiene or vitamin deficiency. Herpes simplex is a viral infection which causes the familiar "cold sore." The herpes lesion is a cluster of small blisters which erupt and crust over. Syphilitic chancre can be found about the mouth. The primary lesion has an indurated button-like appearance.

5. (b) Examination of the mouth and gums for signs of irritation from dentures or disease necessitates the removal of dentures. Because the mouth harbors bacteria, it is strongly advisable to always wear gloves when handling dentures or palpating the mouth.

6. (c) Yeast infection (*Candida*, thrush) is characterized by white, curdlike patches on the buccal mucosa. Canker scores (aphthous ulcers) are painful white, round or oval ulcers surrounded by a ring of reddened mucosa. Nontender yellow or white spots on the cheeks, tongue or lips are sebaceous cysts called Fordyce spots and are harmless.

7. (a) Reddened, swollen gum margins characterize inflammation of the gums, or gingivitis. A brownish melanin pigmentation of the gums is normal in dark-skinned persons. Periodontitis results when gingivitis is untreated and the infection spreads to

the deeper gum tissues around the teeth. Periodontitis is a common cause of tooth loss.

8. (b) The teeth are examined for the following: number present or absent, shape, alignment and relationship to the gums, looseness and tenderness and dental hygiene (caries, fillings, crowns) as well as color (nicotine stains, fluoride pits, dead teeth).

9. (b) Congenital syphilis interferes with the development of the permanent teeth, causing the two upper central incisors to become cone-shaped and notched. Dental caries appear as chalky white deposits on the enamel. As caries progress, they become discolored, and cavities form. Dietary deficiencies result in imperfect dentition or decayed teeth.

10. (c) Most people have a thin, whitish coating on the tongue which is not considered abnormal. Vitamin C deficiency (scurvy) causes swelling, tenderness and hemorrhage of the gums. Leukoplakia refers to white patches on the tongue or mucosa which are not readily scraped off and may be premalignant.

11. (b) Deficiency in vitamin B_{12} or the inability to absorb it due to gastric atrophy (pernicious anemia) results in a smooth, dry, red tongue. Niacin (nicotinic acid) and riboflavin (vitamin B_2) will also produce a sore, reddened tongue. Fungal infection (*Aspergillus niger*) may occur secondarily to antibiotic treatment which inhibits the growth of normal bacterial flora; this is sometimes called black or hairy tongue. With generalized dehydration, the tongue develops longitudinal furrows from reduction of the volume of the tongue.

12. (b) Paralysis of the vagus nerve results in failure of the soft palate to rise on the paralyzed side so that the uvula deviates to the unaffected side.

CLINICAL COMPONENT

The Clinical Component for Units 7 through 11 is presented in Unit 12, Head and Neck: Clinical Component. Preview the Clinical Objectives in that unit and the Performance Guide cards for Unit 12 in Appendix II. Facilitate your learning by practicing these skills before proceeding to the next unit.

Name_______________________________

Date_______________________________

PRE-TEST

UNIT 11

1. Lymphatics from the thorax drain up to the supraclavicular nodes.
   a) True
   b) False

2. Weakness of the trapezius and sternocleidomastoid muscles can be caused by paralysis

   of the____C____cranial nerve(s).
   a) XII
   b) VII
   c) XI
   d) IX and X

3. Shortening of the sternocleidomastoid muscle is a condition called
   a) lymphoma.
   b) goiter.
   c) torticollis
   d) mastoiditis.

4. Swallowing causes the lateral parts of the thyroid tissue to____C____against the examiner's fingers.
   a) fall
   b) remain stationary
   c) rise

5. Malignant nodules are usually tender to palpation.
   a) True
   b) False

6. The trachea is inspected and palpated for deviation and mobility.
   a) True
   b) False

7. The thyroid may be palpated from either the front or back of the client.
   a) True
   b) False

8. If the thyroid is enlarged, the examiner should auscultate the lateral lobes for a
   a) hum.
   b) bruit.
   c) murmur.

9. Tracheal deviation can result from
   1. pleural or pulmonary problems.
   2. masses in the neck.

3. partial obstruction of the trachea.
a) 1, 2, and 3 are correct.
b) 2 only is correct.
c) 1 and 3 are correct.
d) 2 and 3 are correct.
e) 1 and 2 are correct.

10. Lymph nodes are always palpable but not often observable.
a) True
b) False

11. Enlargement of the lymph nodes is termed
a) lymphogonia.
b) lymphoma.
c) lymphadenitis.
d) lymphadenopathy.

Indicate the location of the structures in 12 through 14 in the accompanying diagram.

12. ___B___ Thyroid cartilage

13. ___D___ Thyroid gland

14. ___C___ Cricoid cartilage

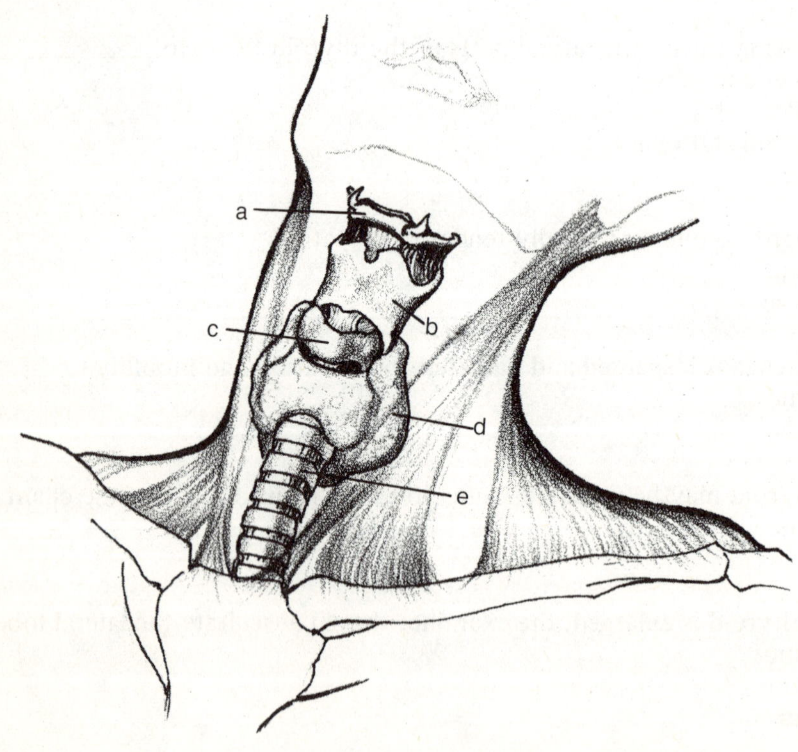

Indicate the location of the structures in 15 through 20 in the following diagram.

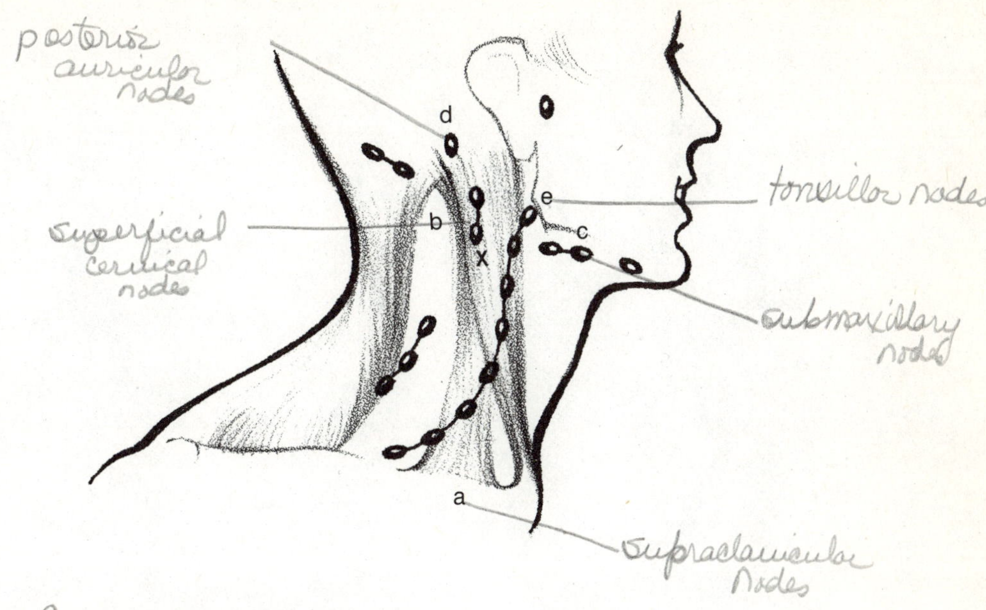

15. __A__   Supraclavicular nodes

16. __B__   Superficial cervical nodes

17. __C__   Submaxillary nodes

18. __E__   Tonsillar nodes

19. __D__   Posterior auricular nodes

20. The muscle labeled "X" is the
    a) sternocleidomastoid muscle.
    b) trapezius muscle.
    c) omohyoid muscle.

Number 11
Examination of the Neck and Lymph Glands

RATIONALE

The purpose of this self-instructional unit is to help you learn inspection, palpation and auscultation of the structures of the neck and associated lymph nodes. This unit concentrates on identifying and describing normal structures and function. Some common abnormal findings are also included. At the end of this unit you will be able to perform an examination of the neck, describe your findings and differentiate between normal and abnormal features.

GLOSSARY OF TERMS

Review the following terms before and after completing this unit. You should be able to define or describe them readily.

Bruit *a murmur or other sound related to circulation, heard over a part*

Goiter *enlargement of the thyroid gland.*

Hodgkin's disease *a malignant lymphoma*

Hypertrophic *pertaining to an increase in size of an organ due to enlargement of its constituent cells.*

Lymphadenitis *inflammation of the lymph nodes*

Lymphadenopathy *enlargement or disease of the lymph nodes.*

Lymphadenosis *hyperplasia or neoplasia affecting the lymph nodes*

Lymphoma *any neoplasm, usually malignant, of lymphatic tissues*

Leukemia *uncontrolled proliferation of leukocytes*

Preauricular, postauricular *in front of (behind) the ear*

Suboccipital *below the occipital bone*

Submaxillary *below the maxilla*

Submental _under the skin_

Supraclavicular _above the clavicle_

Torticollis _deformity of the neck due to contraction of the cervical muscles or sternocleidamastoid_

COGNITIVE OBJECTIVES

At the end of the unit you will demonstrate knowledge of inspection and palpation of the neck and lymph glands by your ability to:

1. Systematically list or label the structures of the neck evaluated during the physical examination and describe normal findings for each: lymph nodes, trachea, thyroid, neck muscles.

2. Describe the features of abnormal lymph nodes and name causative conditions.

3. Discuss conditions that cause tracheal deviation.

4. Describe the procedure for determining characteristics of the thyroid gland.

5. Describe testing for patency of cranial nerves innervating the neck and relate normal responses.

6. Discuss signs and symptoms which could indicate dysfunction.

LEARNING ACTIVITIES

The Learning Activities contain the information necessary for meeting the Cognitive Objectives. Select one and work with it until you have mastered the material. Use the Cognitive Objectives as a study guide. A Self-Test is provided so that you can check how much you know. If you have difficulty with the Self-Test, please review the material in this unit.

Reading Activities

a) Bates: *A Guide to Physical Examination*. Read pp. 28–29 for a description of the anatomy of the neck musculature, cartilaginous structures, vessels and lymph nodes; pp. 45–47 for inspection, palpation and some abnormal findings; p. 72 for examples of thyroid and nodule enlargement; and p. 275 for evaluation of XI cranial nerve.

b) DeGowin and DeGowin: *Bedside Diagnostic Examination*. Detailed descriptions of anatomy and examination techniques and findings are presented. Key signs and symptoms are emphasized. This text is geared for the more advanced practitioner.

c) Delp and Manning: *Major's Physical Diagnosis*, Chapter 4, "Examination of the Head and Neck." This reading gives a brief overview of the examination procedure. Palpation of the thyroid gland is well explained. Extensive supplementation will be necessary for meeting the Cognitive Objectives. Excellent photographs of abnormalities are included.

d) Gillies and Alyn: *Patient Assessment and Management by the Nurse Practitioner*, pp. 58–63. Knowledge of anatomical location of neck structures is assumed. Step-by-step examination of the lymph nodes, thyroid gland and trachea is explained. Normal findings are stressed.

e) Judge and Zuidema: *Methods of Clinical Examination: A Physiological Approach*. Information about the neck and lymph nodes is integrated throughout the text.

f) Prior and Silberstein: *Physical Diagnosis*, Chapter 6, "Head, Face and Neck," pp. 71–77. This section offers a comprehensive coverage of inspection and palpation of the lymph glands, trachea and thyroid gland. Knowledge of anatomy is assumed.

g) Sana and Judge: *Physical Appraisal Methods in Nursing Practice*. Information about the neck and lymph is integrated throughout the text.

h) Sherman and Fields: *Guide to Patient Evaluation*, Chapter 8, pp. 63, 66–71. This chapter provides a brief description of inspection and palpation of the neck, with the emphasis on normal findings. It provides a good introductory reading.

Audiovisual Activities

a) Blue-Hill Educational Systems, Inc.: "Neck – Part 8" and "Nodes – Part 9" (video tape programs). These two programs cover the normal and abnormal findings associated with inspection, palpation and auscultation of the neck. Emphasis is on detecting deviations in symmetry, tracheal position and thyroid and nodal enlargement. Identification and description of masses are well covered. A brief demonstration of examination of the neck and nodes is also included.

Supplemental Activity

The following is suggested to supplement or strengthen your learning.

a) Mechner, Francis: "Patient Assessment: Examination of the Head and Neck." *AJN*, Vol. 75, No. 5, May 1975 (programmed instruction).

SELF-TEST

This Self-Test is for you. Use it to check how well you have learned the material presented in the unit. The answers follow the test.

1. Name the lymph nodes diagrammed in the accompanying illustration.

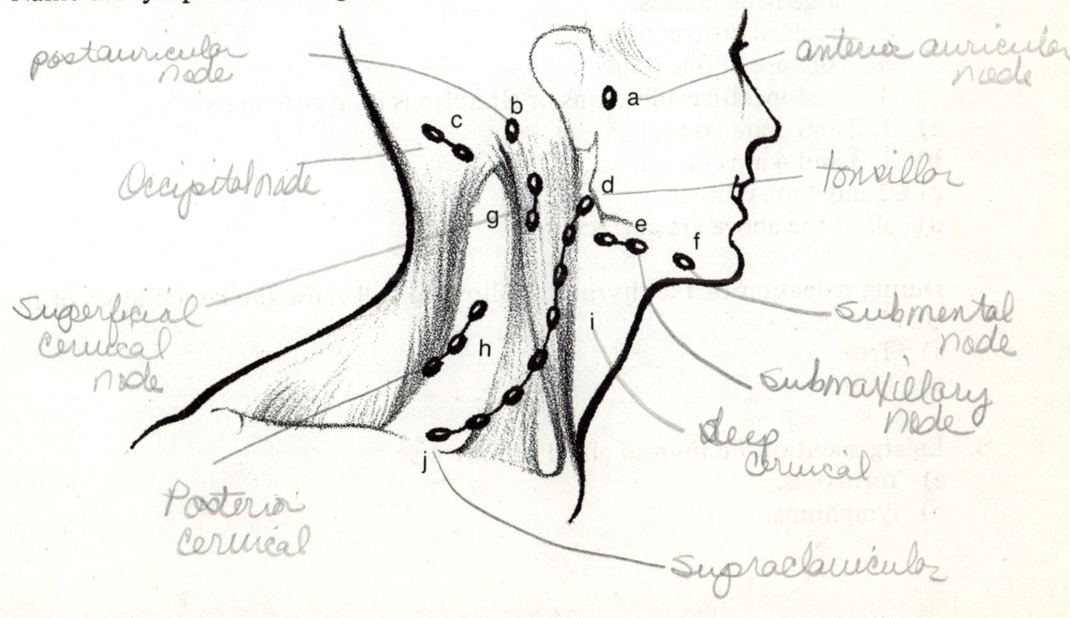

a) _preauricular_ f) _submaxillary_

b) _postauricular_ g) _superficial cervical_

c) _occipital_ h) _posterior cervical_

d) _tonsillar_ i) _deep cervical_

e) _submental_ j) _suprascapular_

2. Identify the following structures using the labels on the accompanying drawing.

_B_ Thyroid cartilage

_C_ Cricoid cartilage

_D_ Thyroid gland

_E_ Trachea

_A_ Hyoid bone

3. Tender lymph nodes generally suggest
   a) inflammation.
   b) malignancy.

4. The supraclavicular nodes receive lymphatic drainage from
   neck, head, abdomen, breast, thorax, arms .

5. The _sternocleidomastoid_ muscle overlies the deep cervical lymph node chain.

6. The examiner may observe or palpate tracheal deviation due to
   1. large neck masses.
   2. tracheal obstruction.
   3. collapse of one lung.
   4. postoperative adhesions or alterations in muscle mass.
   a) 1, 2 and 3 are correct.
   b) 1, 3 and 4 are correct.
   c) 2 and 4 are correct.
   d) all of the above are correct.

7. During palpation of the thyroid, swallowing will cause the lateral lobes of the thyroid gland to rise.
   a) True
   b) False

8. Enlargement of the thyroid gland is known as
   a) torticollis.
   b) lymphoma.

   c) goiter.
   d) lymphadenitis.
   e) gout.

9. Neck and shoulder muscles are innervated by the _____*A*_____ cranial nerve.
   a) XI (spinal accessory)
   b) XII (hypoglossal)
   c) IX (glossopharyngeal)
   d) V (trigeminal)

SELF-TEST KEY

1. (a) preauricular   (f) submental
   (b) posterior auricular   (g) superficial cervical
   (c) occipital   (h) posterior cervical chain
   (d) tonsillar   (i) deep cervical chain
   (e) submaxillary   (j) supraclavicular

2. (b) thyroid cartilage
   (c) cricoid cartilage
   (d) thyroid gland
   (e) trachea
   (a) hyoid bone.

3. (a) With inflammation the lymph nodes tend to become enlarged and tender. In cases of malignancy, the nodes are most often stony hard and nontender.

4. Lymph drains from the head and neck to the supraclavicular nodes. These nodes also receive drainage from the abdomen, breasts, thorax and arms.

5. The sternocleidomastoid muscle overlies most of the deep cervical lymph node chain except for the tonsillar and supraclavicular nodes which are most often palpable.

6. (b) Masses, adhesions or surgical alterations of tissue in the neck may displace the normal midline position of the trachea. Alterations in normal intrathoracic pressures, as occur with collapse of the lung, will result in deviation of the trachea. Tracheal obstruction will not alter its midline position.

7. (a) During swallowing, the trachea and thyroid rise. Structures such as masses and lymph nodes do not rise.

8. (c) Goiter due to iodine deficiency results in an enlarged thyroid gland. Lymphoma is a general term for a neoplasm of the lymphatic system. Lymphadenitis is an inflammation of the lymph gland. Gout is a painful condition in which urate crystals are deposited in the cartilage of joints, usually the big toe.

9. (a) The spinal accessory cranial nerve innervates the shoulder and neck muscles which enable the movements of shrugging the shoulders and turning the head. The hypoglossal nerve supplies motor fibers to the tongue. The glossopharyngeal innervates the tongue and pharynx. The muscles of the jaw are supplied by the trigeminal nerve.

CLINICAL COMPONENT

The Clinical Component for Units 7 through 11 is presented in Unit 12, Head and Neck: Clinical Component. Preview the Clinical Objectives in that unit and the Performance Guide cards for Unit 12 in Appendix II. Facilitate your learning by practicing these skills before proceeding to the next unit.

Number 12

Head and Neck:
Clinical Component

Having completed Units 7 through 11, you are now ready to proceed with the Clinical Objectives. The purpose of this Clinical Component is to help you learn to assess the head and neck for normal configuration and to detect the presence, location and extent of any abnormalities.

CLINICAL OBJECTIVES

At the end of this unit you will perform systematic assessment of the head and neck, correlating physical examination skills with physiological principles. You will be able to:

1. Demonstrate knowledge of signs and symptoms of dysfunction related to the head and neck by obtaining a pertinent health history from a client.

2. Demonstrate inspection of the eye by
   a. assessing the external structures of the eye.
   b. utilizing the Snellen chart to test visual acuity.
   c. grossly testing visual fields.
   d. testing extraocular movements.
   e. checking for strabismus with the cover test.

3. Demonstrate and correctly interpret Weber and Rinne tests.

4. Demonstrate inspection and palpation of the ear by
   a. assessing and describing the external structures of the ear and mastoid process.
   b. utilizing the otoscope to systematically describe the external auditory canal, landmarks of the tympanic membrane and patency of the eustachian tube.

5. Demonstrate inspection of the nose by
   a. identifying and describing the external features of the nose.
   b. utilizing an otoscope and nasal attachment to systematically identify and describe the internal nasal structures.

6. Demonstrate palpation of the frontal and maxillary sinuses.

7. Systematically inspect and describe the structures of the mouth and pharynx.

8. Demonstrate inspection and palpation of the neck by
   a. systematically evaluating the integrity of lymph nodes.
   b. assessing the trachea and thyroid.

9. Demonstrate examination for opacities by eliciting the red reflex (fundus glow) and locating opacities.

10. Demonstrate ophthalmoscopy by
    a. properly preparing the client and environment.
    b. correctly manipulating the ophthalmoscope.
    c. visualizing and systematically describing the disc, vessels, general background and macula.

11. Demonstrate assessment of intraocular pressure by light palpation.

12. Utilize S.O.A.P. to describe findings systematically, make an assessment regarding normality and formulate a plan of action.

INSTRUCTIONS

Utilizing three of your peers or clients in the clinical area, practice inspection and palpation of the head and neck. Remove Performance Guide cards for Unit 12 in Appendix II. These cards will enable you to practice the skills necessary to meet the Clinical Objectives and complete the Response Sheets. On each Response Sheet, you will be expected to (1) ask questions which elicit possible symptoms, (2) systematically describe your findings, (3) localize any abnormalities present and (4) summarize your examination using the S.O.A.P. method of recording.

When you have mastered the Clinical Objectives and completed the Response Sheets arrange to demonstrate your skills to your laboratory instructor or preceptor.

EQUIPMENT

You will need the following equipment to complete the examinations:

    Card for eye cover
    Cotton applicator
    Ophthalmoscope
    Otoscope with ear and nasal specula
    Plastic gloves
    Small flashlight
    Snellen chart
    Tongue blades
    Tuning fork
    Taste and smell testing condiments

OPTIONAL ACTIVITIES

These activities demonstrate examination techniques of the head and neck assessment.
a) Bates: "Head and Neck" (film).
b) Blue-Hill Educational Systems, Inc.: "Head and Neck" (18 minutes), "Ear, Nose, Throat and Mouth (19 minutes) and "Eyes" (45 minutes) (video tape).

RESPONSE SHEET—HEAD AND NECK

Client _______________________________

Date_______________________ Age ________ Sex_______

Examiner_______________________________

I. Health History

II. Physical Examination (Describe findings; diagram abnormalities)

A. Eyes

    1. Visual acuity:

    2. Visual fields:

    3. External eye:

        a. General

        b. Lids

        c. Ducts

        d. Conjunctiva

        e. Sclera

        f. Cornea/lens

    g. Iris

    h. Pupils

  4. EOM's

B. Ophthalmoscopy

  1. Opacities

  2. Disc

  3. Vessels

  4. General background

  5. Macula

  6. Intraocular tension

C. Ears

  1. External

    a. Pinna

    b. Mastoid

  2. Otoscopic canal

    a. Canal

    b. Tympanic membrane

3. Auditory acuity

D. Nose

1. External

2. Internal

3. Sinuses

4. Smell

E. Mouth and Pharynx

1. Mouth

a. Lips

b. Mucosa

c. Gums

d. Teeth

e. Ducts

f. Hard palate

g. Tongue

2. Pharynx

a. Uvula

    b. Soft palate

    c. Pillars

    d. Tonsils

    e. Posterior pharynx

  3. Taste

F. Neck

  1. General

  2. Lymph nodes

  3. Trachea

  4. Thyroid

  5. Trapezius and sternocleidomastoid muscles

Summarize your findings using the S.O.A.P. method.

S. **(Client's observations, complaints, health history)**

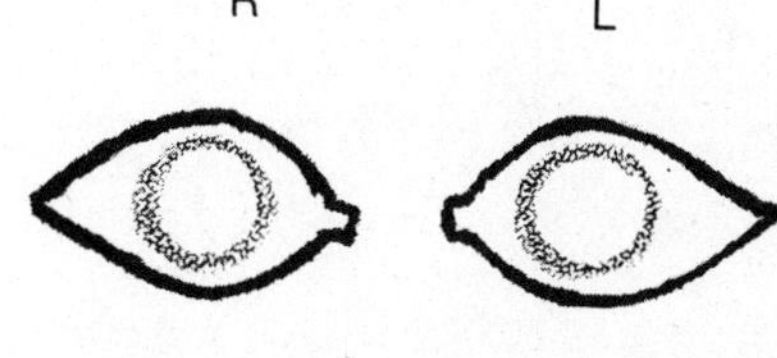

O. **(Physical findings)**

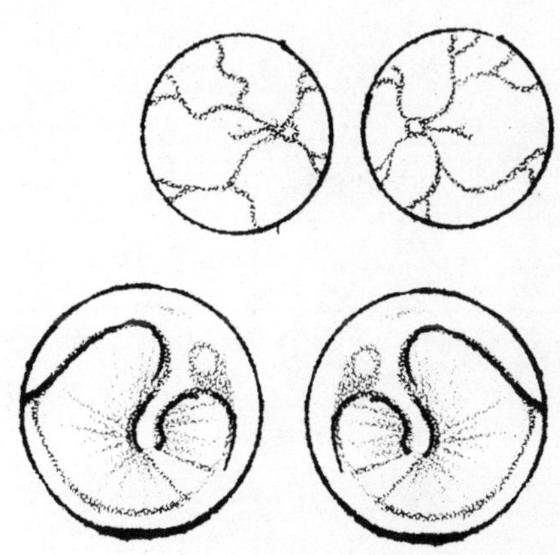

A. **(Assessment of problem, data, prognosis)**

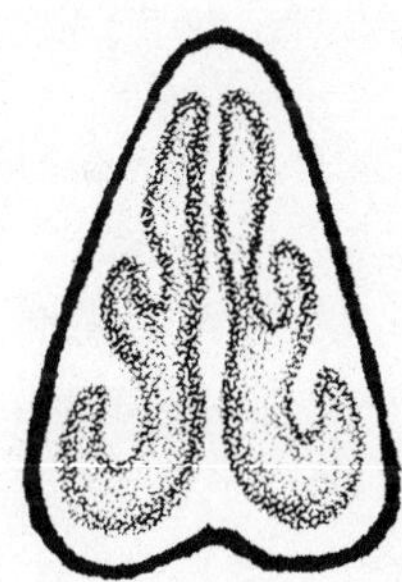

P. **(Plans for further evaluation, care, teaching)**

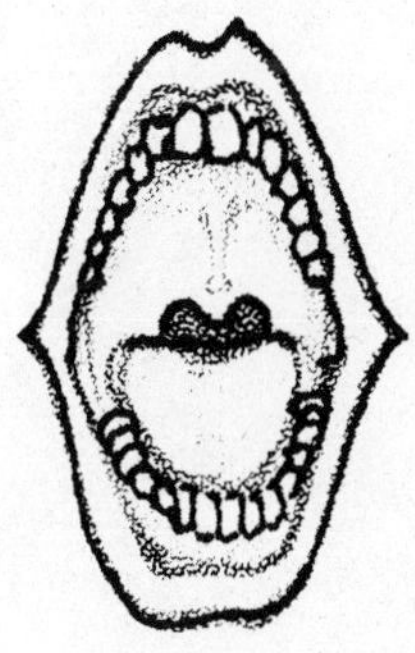

RESPONSE SHEET—HEAD AND NECK

Client _______________________________________

Date _________________________ Age _______ Sex _____

Examiner ____________________________________

I. Health History

II. Physical Examination (Describe findings; diagram abnormalities)

A. Eyes

1. Visual acuity:

2. Visual fields:

3. External eye:

   a. General

   b. Lids

   c. Ducts

   d. Conjunctiva

   e. Sclera

   f. Cornea/lens

    g. Iris

    h. Pupils

  4. EOM's

B. Ophthalmoscopy

  1. Opacities

  2. Disc

  3. Vessels

  4. General background

  5. Macula

  6. Intraocular tension

C. Ears

  1. External

    a. Pinna

    b. Mastoid

  2. Otoscopic canal

    a. Canal

    b. Tympanic membrane

3. Auditory acuity

D. Nose

1. External

2. Internal

3. Sinuses

4. Smell

E. Mouth and Pharynx

1. Mouth

a. Lips

b. Mucosa

c. Gums

d. Teeth

e. Ducts

f. Hard palate

g. Tongue

2. Pharynx

a. Uvula

    b. Soft palate

    c. Pillars

    d. Tonsils

    e. Posterior pharynx

3. Taste

F. Neck

1. General

2. Lymph nodes

3. Trachea

4. Thyroid

5. Trapezius and sternocleidomastoid muscles

Summarize your findings using the S.O.A.P. method.

S.   **(Client's observations, complaints, health history)**

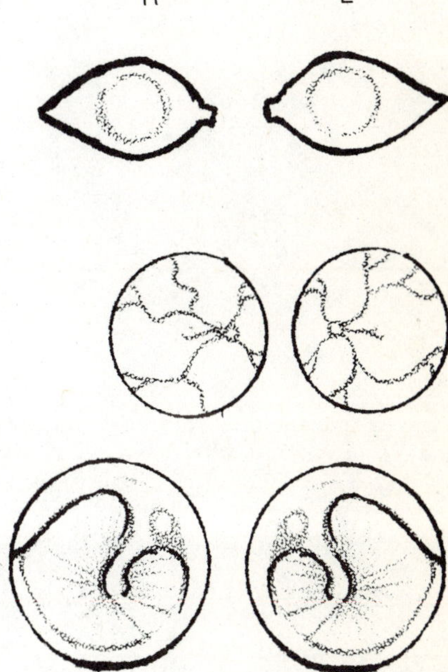

O.   **(Physical findings)**

A.   **(Assessment of problem, data, prognosis)**

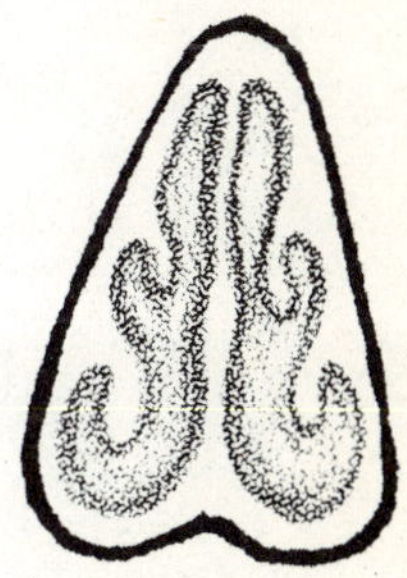

P.   **(Plans for further evaluation, care, teaching)**

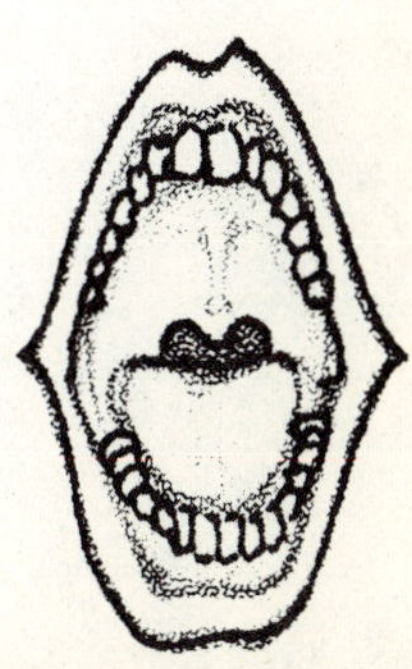

RESPONSE SHEET—HEAD AND NECK

Client _______________________________

Date_________________ Age _______ Sex______

Examiner_______________________________

I. Health History

II. Physical Examination (Describe findings; diagram abnormalities)

A. Eyes

1. Visual acuity:

2. Visual fields:

3. External eye:

    a. General

    b. Lids

    c. Ducts

    d. Conjunctiva

    e. Sclera

    f. Cornea/lens

    g. Iris

    h. Pupils

  4. EOM's

B. Ophthalmoscopy

  1. Opacities

  2. Disc

  3. Vessels

  4. General background

  5. Macula

  6. Intraocular tension

C. Ears

  1. External

    a. Pinna

    b. Mastoid

  2. Otoscopic canal

    a. Canal

    b. Tympanic membrane

3. Auditory acuity

D. Nose

1. External

2. Internal

3. Sinuses

4. Smell

E. Mouth and Pharynx

1. Mouth

    a. Lips

    b. Mucosa

    c. Gums

    d. Teeth

    e. Ducts

    f. Hard palate

    g. Tongue

2. Pharynx

    a. Uvula

    b. Soft palate

    c. Pillars

    d. Tonsils

    e. Posterior pharynx

3. Taste

F. Neck

1. General

2. Lymph nodes

3. Trachea

4. Thyroid

5. Trapezius and sternocleidomastoid muscles

Summarize your findings using the S.O.A.P. method.

S. **(Client's observations, complaints, health history)**

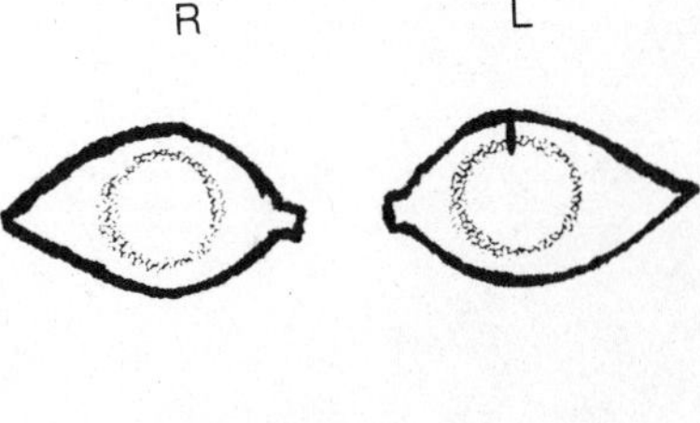

O. **(Physical findings)**

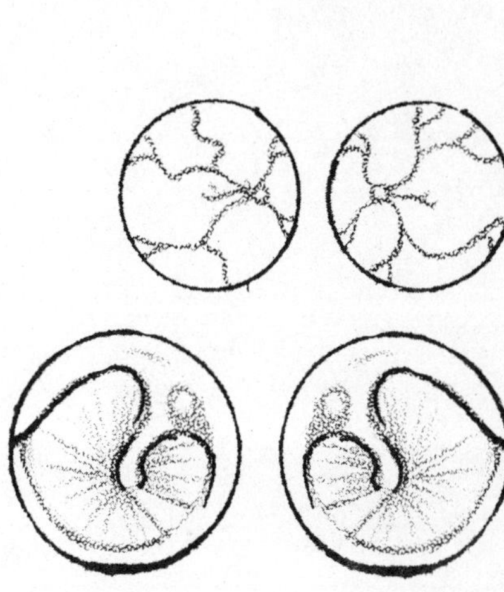

A. **(Assessment of problem, data, prognosis)**

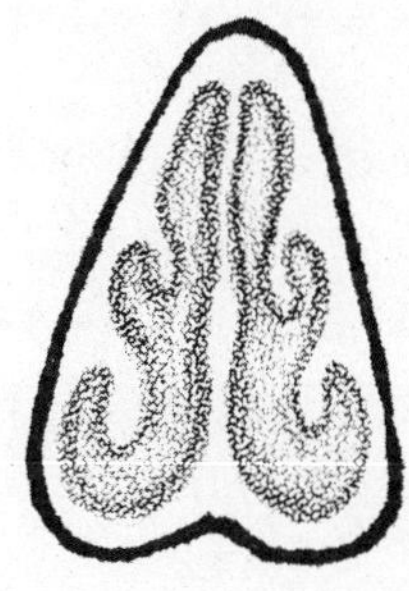

P. **(Plans for further evaluation, care, teaching)**

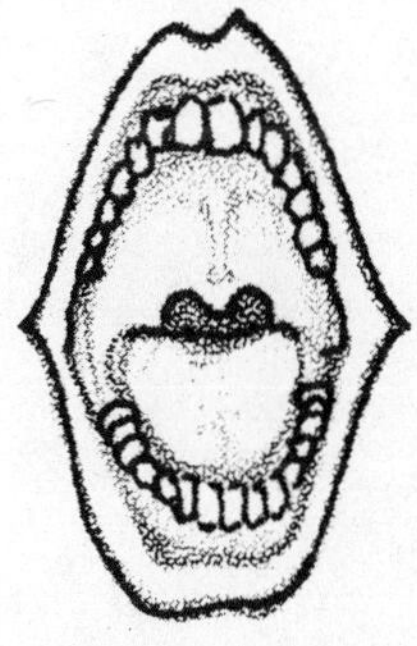

SECTION III

UPPER TORSO

PRE-TEST

UNIT 13

1. Inspection of the breast includes observing
     1. symmetry.
     2. skin tone.
     3. position and size.
     4. amount and color of discharge after stripping the nipple.
     5. dimpling or skin retraction.
   a) 1, 2 and 4 are correct.
   b) 1, 2, 3 and 4 are correct.
   c) 2, 4 and 5 are correct.
   d) 1, 2, 3, and 5 are correct.

2. Nipple inversion is
   a) always indicative of a slow growing neoplasm.
   b) significant only if it is recent.
   c) a rare occurrence.
   d) usually unilateral.

3. Milk-producing structures in the breast are known as
   a) tubercles of Montgomery.
   b) areolae.
   c) acini.
   d) striae.

4. Most lymphatic drainage from the breast is to the node in the
   a) opposite breast.
   b) supraclavicular area.
   c) subscapular area.
   d) axillary area.
   e) mediastinal area.

5. The major components of breast tissue are
     1. fat.
     2. glandular tissue.
     3. fibrous or connective tissue.
     4. striated muscle fibers.
   a) 1, 2 and 4 are correct.
   b) 1, 2 and 3 are correct.
   c) 3 and 4 are correct.
   d) 2 only is correct.
   e) all of the above are correct.

6. Gynecomastia refers to
   a) breast enlargement in men.
   b) breast carcinoma.

     c) cystic disease.
     d) supernumerary breasts.

7. Premenstrual changes in the breasts result in
    a) engorgement.
    b) a lobular feeling which may be confused with masses.
    c) low sensitivity to palpation (this is a good time to examine breasts).
    d) a and b.
    e) b and c.

8. Examination of the breast should be performed with the client
    a) seated.
    b) in a supine position.
    c) in both of the above positions.

9. The lymph nodes most often palpated are the
    a) posterior axillary nodes.
    b) central axillary nodes.
    c) anterior axillary nodes.
    d) supraclavicular lymph nodes.

10. Breast self-examination
      1. is not necessary after menopause.
      2. includes observing in a mirror for puckering of skin and any changes in size, symmetry or contour.
      3. should be performed following each menstrual period or monthly if the client is menopausal.
      4. includes palpating each breast and axilla for nodules while the client is in a reclining position.
    a) all of the above are correct.
    b) 1 and 2 are correct.
    c) 2, 3 and 4 are correct.
    d) 3 only is correct.

Match the following columns (letters may be used more than once).

11. ________ Increased venous prominence

12. ________ Very mobile, nontender, well-delineated mass

13. ________ Recent nipple inversion

14. ________ Soft, round, well-delineated tender masses

15. ________ Ulceration of the nipple

a) Paget's disease
b) Cystic disease
c) Carcinoma
d) Fibroadenoma

16. A young, lactating woman comes to the clinic complaining of a painful right breast. Her temperature is elevated, and she is diaphoretic. The breast is red, hot and swollen. The axillary nodes are not enlarged or tender. You suspect
    a) carcinoma.
    b) trauma.
    c) mastitis.
    d) Paget's disease.

17. A sign of intraductal papilloma is
    a) edema of the breast.
    b) flattening of the nipple.
    c) an increased venous prominence over the breasts.
    d) a bloody discharge from the nipple.
    e) ulceration of the nipple.

18. Visible signs of breast cancer include
    1. dimpling or retraction.
    2. change in breast contour.
    3. nipple deviation.
    4. recent nipple inversion or flattening.
    a) 1 and 3 are correct.
    b) 2 only is correct.
    c) 1, 3 and 4 are correct.
    d) all of the above are correct.

19. A *peau d'orange* sign is found in
    a) intraductal papilloma.
    b) lymphatic blockage.
    c) Paget's disease.
    d) hyperpigmentation.
    e) gynecomastia.

20. The characteristics of a malignant breast tumor include
    1. soft, smooth surface.
    2. firm, uneven surface.
    3. well-defined border.
    4. irregular margins.
    5. easily movable mass.
    6. mass often fixed to underlying tissue.
    a) 1, 3 and 5 are correct.
    b) 2, 4 and 5 are correct.
    c) 2, 4 and 6 are correct.
    d) 1, 4 and 6 are correct.
    e) 2, 3 and 5 are correct.

Number 13
Examination of the Breasts and Axillae

RATIONALE

This self-instructional unit is designed to help you learn systematic inspection and palpation of the breasts. Focus is on examination techniques, normal findings, common abnormalities and utilizing breast self-examinations as a method of early cancer detection. At the end of this unit you will be able to inspect breast tissue for normal configuration; palpate both breasts and axillae for consistency, tenderness or nodules; and teach breast self-examination to a client or peer.

GLOSSARY OF TERMS

Review the following terms before and after completing this unit. You should be able to define or describe them readily.

Acini ____

Areola ____

Colostrum ____

Cooper's ligaments ____

Erythema ____

Fibroadenoma ____

Gynecomastia ____

Intraductal papilloma ____

Mastitis ____

Paget's disease ____

Striae ____

Supernumerary breasts ____

Tubercles of Montgomery
 (Montgomery's follicles) ____

COGNITIVE OBJECTIVES

At the end of this unit you will demonstrate knowledge of inspection and palpation of the breasts and axillae by your ability to:

1. Correctly identify or diagram the anatomy of the breast, axillary lymph nodes and direction of lymph flow from the breast.

2. Systematically list all the structures inspected and palpated during breast examination.
   a. Describe examination procedure for each structure.
   b. Describe normal findings for each area.
   c. Differentiate between male and female examination procedures and findings.

3. Discuss signs and symptoms of dysfunction associated with common abnormalities: gynecomastia, mastitis, Paget's disease, adenofibromas, malignant neoplasms, cystic disease, intraductal papilloma, supernumerary breasts.

4. Explain the importance of monthly breast self-examination.
   a. Describe observations and procedure.
   b. Discuss possible limiting or facilitating factors.

LEARNING ACTIVITIES

The Learning Activities contain the information necessary for meeting the Cognitive Objectives. Select one and proceed to work with it until you have mastered the material. Use the Cognitive Objectives as a study guide. A Self-Test is provided so that you can check how much you know. If you have difficulty with the Self-Test, please review the material in this unit before proceeding to the Clinical Objectives.

At the end of this unit you will complete the Clinical Component. Preview the Clinical Objectives and the Performance Guide cards for Unit 13 in Appendix II for inspection and palpation of the breast and axillae.

Reading Activities

a) Bates: *A Guide to Physical Examination*, "The Breasts and Axillae." The reading reviews anatomy and physiology of breasts and axillae, examination procedures and normal and abnormal findings. This chapter is exceptionally well illustrated. Guidelines for teaching breast self-examination are not presented.

b) Delp and Manning: *Major's Physical Diagnosis*, "Examination of the Breast." Student's knowledge of anatomy of breasts and axillae is assumed. Examination procedures and abnormalities are described and accompanied by many photographs. Normal breast findings and principles of breast self-examination are not discussed.

c) DeGowin and DeGowin: *Bedside Diagnostic Examination*, "The Breasts." The anatomy of the breasts and lymph nodes is reviewed. Examination procedures are outlined thoroughly and illustrated. Signs and symptoms of dysfunction are emphasized. Additional reading will be necessary to identify normal findings and principles of breast self-examination.

d) Gillies and Alyn: *Patient Assessment and Management by the Nurse Practitioner*, "Examination of the Breasts," pp. 63–67. A fairly comprehensive overview of breast examination is presented. Abnormal findings are discussed and related to possible disorders. The student will need to review other readings for anatomy of the breasts and axillae, normal findings and techniques of breast self-examination.

e) Judge and Zuidema: *Methods of Clinical Examination: A Physiologic Approach*, "The Breast." Anatomy of breasts and axillae, normal findings, signs and symptoms of dysfunction and guidelines for teaching breast self-examination are clearly and concisely presented in this chapter.

f) Prior and Silberstein: *Physical Diagnosis*, "The Breast." This chapter presents information in a very readable format. Essential information is presented with the exclusion of anatomy review and techniques of breast self-examination. Diagrams and photographs are used extensively to illustrate the text.

g) Sana and Judge: *Physical Appraisal Methods in Nursing Practice*, "Physical Appraisal of the Female Reproductive System," pp. 230–239. Comprehensive discussion of procedures of breast and axillary examination. Normal findings and importance of self-examination are stressed. Abnormal signs and symptoms are related to possible disease states. The student who is unfamiliar with anatomical structures of the breasts and axillae will need to refer to another text.

h) Sherman and Fields: *Guide to Patient Evaluation*, "The Breasts." This chapter presents an overview of anatomy and physiology of the breast, but not of the lymph nodes. Examination techniques, normal features and some abnormal findings for both female and male breasts are discussed. Techniques of breast self-examination are not covered in this well-illustrated chapter.

Audiovisual Activities

a) Blue-Hill Educational Systems, Inc.: "The Breasts," Tape X. This program presents a systematic approach to examining the breasts, nipples and associated lymph nodes, contrasting normal and abnormal findings. The epidemiology of breast cancer is also discussed. A cursory examination is demonstrated, using the "Betsi" model. Anatomy and physiology of the breast should be reviewed before viewing this video tape presentation.

b) Ortho Pharmaceutical Co. OMNI series: "Breast Examination." This series consists of four programmed instruction booklets which extensively cover (1) anatomy and physiology, (2) examination procedures, (3) description and classification of findings and (4) breast self-examination. Slide-tape and video tape cassette activities accompany the booklets.

Supplemental Activities

The following materials are suggested to supplement or strengthen your learning.

a) Cohen, Frederick B., Cooper, Richard G., and Mitchell, Malcolm S.: "Managing Cancer with Chemotherapy." *Nursing Update*, Vol. 6, No. 12, December 1975.

b) Egan, Robert L., et al.: "A Nursing Guide to Breast Cancer Prevention." *Nursing Update*, Vol. 6, No. 11, November 1975.

SELF-TEST

This Self-Test is for you. Use it to check how well you have learned the material presented in the unit. The answers follow the test.

1. Identify the structures in the following drawing.

a) ______________________________

b) ______________________________

c) ______________________________

d) ______________________________

e) ______________________________

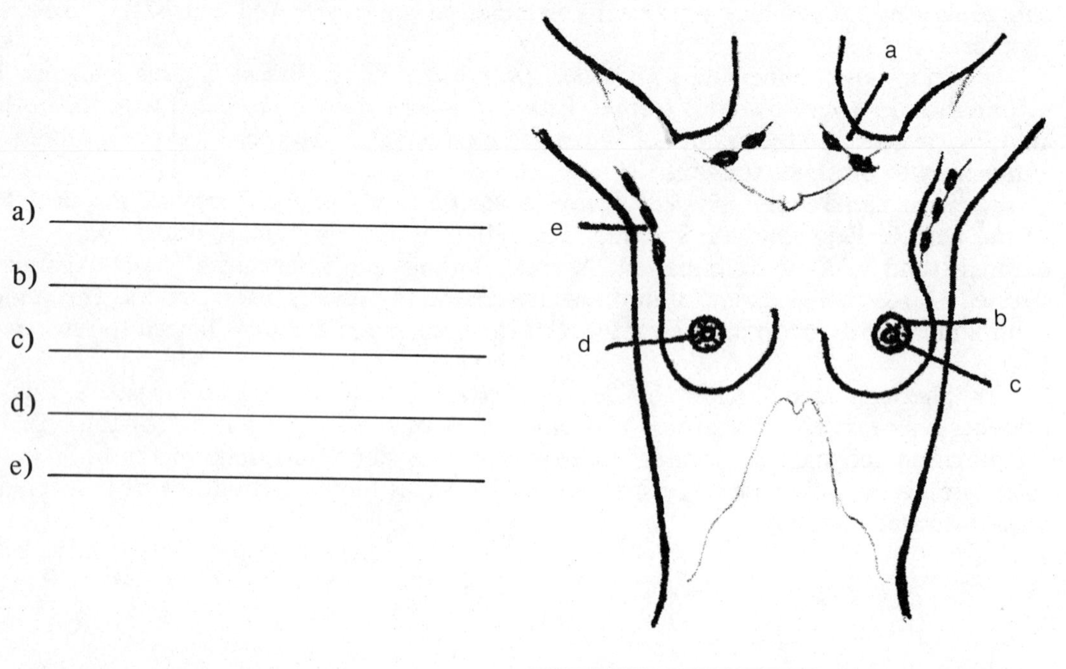

2. The breasts are inspected for
    a) symmetry.
    b) position and size.
    c) skin retraction.
    d) all of the above.

3. To bring out dimpling or retraction of the breast or nipples you should
    a) ask the client to raise her hands over her head.
    b) instruct the client to bend forward to bring the breasts away from the chest wall.
    c) strip the nipple.
    d) ask the patient to place her hands on her hips and push forcibly against them.
    e) request that the client perform movements in a and d.
    f) have the client perform all of the above except c.

Indicate whether statements 4 through 7 about palpation are True (a) or False (b).

4. ________ The consistency of breast tissue varies very little.

5. ________ Palpation of the breast should be performed with the patient sitting and supine.

6. ________ A very tender and moderately firm breast suggests inflammation.

7. ________ The male breast (areolae and nipples) should also be palpated for nodules.

8. Malignant neoplasms are usually
    1. very hard.
    2. fixed to underlying tissue.
    3. tender.
    4. well-circumscribed.

    a) 1 and 3 are correct.
    b) 2 and 4 are correct.
    c) 1 and 2 are correct.
    d) all of the above are correct.

9. Gynecomastia is
    a) a female breast occurring in a male.
    b) inflammation of the lactating breast.
    c) characterized by excoriation of the nipple.
    d) a firm multilobulated lesion found in young women.

10. List five observable signs of breast cancer.

    a) _______________________________

    b) _______________________________

    c) _______________________________

    d) _______________________________

    e) _______________________________

11. At what time in the menstrual cycle is breast self-examination best performed?

SELF-TEST KEY

1. (a) supraclavicular nodes, (b) areola, (c) nipple, (d) Montgomery's tubercle, (e) central axillary nodes.

2. (d) Inspection of the breasts includes checking symmetry, position and size, skin retraction and the general appearance of the skin and nipples. Some asymmetry in size and position is not uncommon and is usually developmental. Recent changes, however, might indicate an abnormality.

3. (f) Raising the hands above the head and also pushing forcibly on the hips causes contraction of the pectoral muscles and results in a pull on the breast tissue, exaggerating any retraction that may be present. Having the client with large or pendulous breasts lean forward, freeing the breasts from the chest wall may also bring out dimpling or retraction. Stripping may evert a retracted nipple.

4. False. The consistency of breast tissue varies considerably, depending on such factors as age, parity, stage of menstrual cycle, obesity and pregnancy.

5. True. Besides being palpated in the sitting and supine positions, breasts should also be palpated with the client's arm at her side and then with arms overhead.

6. True. Tenderness usually indicates inflammation. Malignant tumors are rarely tender and are usually very firm.

7. True. In the male breast, a hard irregular nodule located behind the areola is indicative of possible neoplasm.

8. (c) Malignant neoplasms are usually nontender, firm, irregular and infiltrating and fixed to underlying tissue.

9. (a) Gynecomastia is a smooth, firm, frequently tender disc of breast tissue which develops behind the areola of the male breast resulting in enlargement. It may be unilateral or bilateral and is not an uncommon phenomenon during puberty. In the older male, gynecomastia may be due to systemic diseases such as cirrhosis of the liver, in which the liver fails to detoxify estrogen.

10. Observations which suggest possible malignancy include dimpling, changes in breast contour, recent flattening or inversion of a nipple, hard, fixed nontender nodules, edema of the breast, and an increased prominence of the venous pattern.

11. Clients should be taught to examine their breasts after the menstrual flow has stopped. Hormonal influences are less apparent, and there is a better opportunity to feel the underlying breast tissue accurately.

CLINICAL COMPONENT

Having completed the cognitive portion of this unit, you are now ready to proceed to the Clinical Objectives. The purpose of the Clinical Component is to assess the breasts and axillae for normal configuration and detect the presence, location and extent of any dysfunction.

CLINICAL OBJECTIVES

At the end of this unit you will be able to perform assessment of breasts and axillae, correlating physical examination skills with physiological principles. You will be able to:

1. Demonstrate knowledge of signs and symptoms of dysfunction related to the breasts and axillae by obtaining a pertinent health history from the client.

2. Demonstrate inspection of the breasts and axillae, with the client in both sitting and supine positions, by systematically assessing
   a. the breasts for size, contour and skin characteristics.
   b. the areolae and nipples for size, shape, direction and skin characteristics.
   c. the axillae for rashes.

3. Demonstrate palpation of the breasts and axillae by systematically assessing
   a. the breasts for consistency, nodules or tenderness.
   b. the nipples for elasticity or discharge.
   c. the axillae for nodules and tenderness.
   d. the supraclavicular area for enlarged lymph nodes.

4. Utilize S.O.A.P. to systematically describe findings, make an assessment regarding normality and formulate a plan of action.

5. Teach breast self-examination to the client or in a role-playing situation.

INSTRUCTIONS

Utilizing three of your peers or clients in the clinical area, practice inspection and palpation of the breasts and axillae. Remove the Performance Guide cards for Unit 13 in Appendix II. These cards will enable you to practice the skills necessary to meet the Clinical Objectives and complete the Response Sheets. On each Response Sheet you will be expected to (1) ask questions which elicit possible symptoms, (2) systematically describe your examination findings, (3) localize any abnormalities present and (4) summarize the examination using the S.O.A.P. method of recording.

Client______________________________

Date________________ Age _______ Sex______

Examiner____________________________

I. Health History

II. Physical Examination

A. Inspection

1. Breasts

2. Areolae and nipples

3. Axillae

B. Palpation

1. Breasts

2. Areolae and nipples

3. Axillae and lymph nodes

Summarize your findings using the S.O.A.P. method.

S.   (Client's observations, complaints, health history)

O.   (Physical findings)
Locate any abnormal findings on the
accompanying diagram.

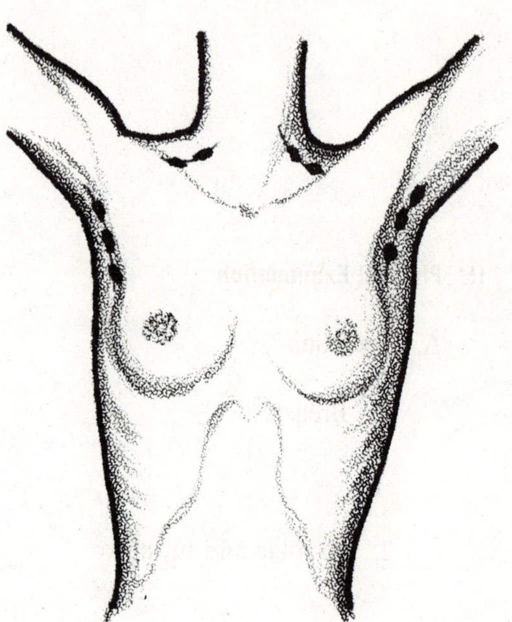

A.   (Assessment of problem, data, prognosis)

P.   (Plans for further evaluation, care, teaching)

Client________________________________

Date__________________ Age ______ Sex______

Examiner________________________________

I. Health History

II. Physical Examination

A. Inspection

   1. Breasts

   2. Areolae and nipples

   3. Axillae

B. Palpation

   1. Breasts

   2. Areolae and nipples

   3. Axillae and lymph nodes

Summarize your findings using the S.O.A.P. method.

S. (Client's observations, complaints, health history)

O. (Physical findings)
Locate any abnormal findings on the
accompanying diagram.

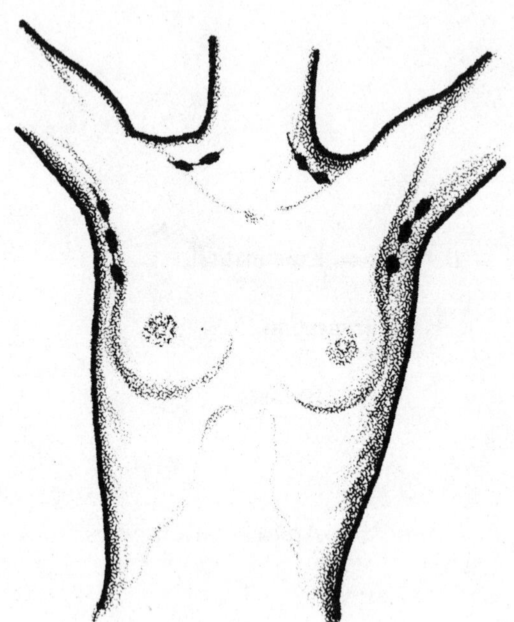

A. (Assessment of problem, data, prognosis)

P. (Plans for further evaluation, care, teaching)

Client ________________________________

Date _________________ Age _______ Sex _______

Examiner _______________________________

I. Health History

II. Physical Examination

A. Inspection

1. Breasts

2. Areolae and nipples

3. Axillae

B. Palpation

1. Breasts

2. Areolae and nipples

3. Axillae and lymph nodes

Summarize your findings using the S.O.A.P. method.

S. **(Client's observations, complaints, health history)**

O. **(Physical findings)**
Locate any abnormal findings on the
accompanying diagram.

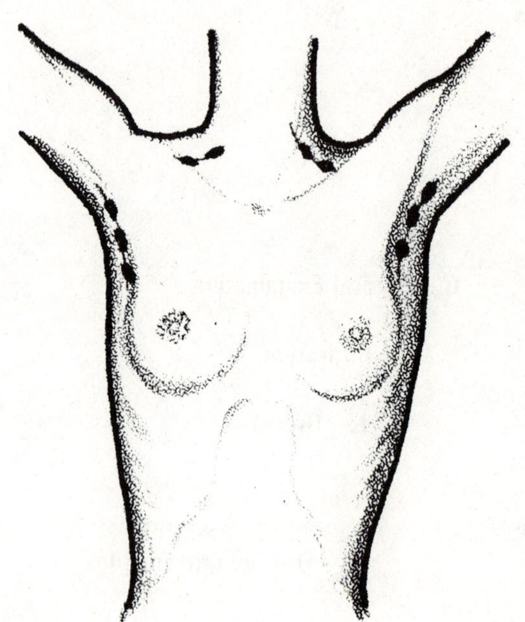

A. **(Assessment of problem, data, prognosis)**

P. **(Plans for further evaluation, care, teaching)**

PRE-TEST

UNIT 14

Mark the statements in 1 through 7 (a) for True or (b) for False.

1. _______ Cheyne-Stokes respirations are marked by periods of apnea, alternating with periods of hyperpnea.

2. _______ Diaphragmatic breathing is characteristic in women.

3. _______ Rapid, deep respirations seen in diabetic coma are called Biot's respirations.

4. _______ The thorax of a patient with emphysema assumes a position similar to that of full inspiration.

5. _______ Symmetry of lateral expansion can be tested by placing one hand on each side of the posterior midthoracic region, asking the client to inhale deeply and noting movement of trunk from midline.

6. _______ In kyphosis, the AP diameter is greater than normal.

7. _______ Fluid in the pleural space usually increases tactile fremitus.

Choose the one best answer.

8. Percussion of the thorax
   1. includes comparison of symmetrical points.
   2. includes perceiving the character of vibrations that can be heard as well as felt.
   3. is a technique of striking the chest wall to determine densities.
   4. requires that the pleximeter be placed horizontally over the rib, not over the intercostal space.
   a) 1, 2 and 3 are correct.
   b) 1 and 3 are correct.
   c) 3 and 4 are correct.
   d) all of the above are correct.

9. Inspection of the thorax includes checking
   1. rate and depth of respirations.
   2. symmetry of chest excursion.
   3. skeletal deformities.
   4. use of accessory musculature.
   a) 1, 2 and 4 are correct.
   b) 1, 2 and 3 are correct.
   c) 1 and 2 are correct.
   d) all of the above are correct.

10. Dyspnea is a symptom in which the client
    1. complains of chest pain.
    2. is aware of difficulty in breathing.
    3. complains of orthopnea.
    4. is comatose.
 a) 1 and 3 are correct.
 b) 2 and 4 are correct.
 c) 2 only is correct.
 d) all of the above are correct.

11. Hyperresonance may be percussed in which of the following?
    1. COPD
    2. Pleural effusion
    3. Atelectasis
    4. Pneumothorax
 a) 1 only is correct.
 b) 2 and 3 are correct.
 c) 1 and 4 are correct.
 d) all of the above are correct.

12. Diaphragmatic excursion is decreased with
    1. emphysema.
    2. pregnancy.
    3. phrenic nerve paralysis.
    4. ascites.
 a) 1 only is correct.
 b) 1 and 2 are correct.
 c) 3 and 4 are correct.
 d) all of the above are correct.

13. Increased fremitus may be palpated in which of the following?
    1. Pneumonia
    2. COPD
    3. Pulmonary edema
    4. Pleural effusion
 a) 1 and 3 are correct.
 b) 2 and 4 are correct.
 c) 1 only is correct.
 d) all of the above are correct.

14. Dullness to percussion is found in
    1. pneumonia.
    2. COPD
    3. pneumothorax.
    4. pulmonary edema.
 a) 1, 3 and 4 are correct.
 b) 2 only is correct.
 c) 1 and 4 are correct.
 d) 1 only is correct.

15. Diaphragmatic excursion is
    1. measured during full inspiration and full expiration.
    2. measured on the anterior chest.

    3. a percussion maneuver.
    4. greater in men than women.
a) 1 and 4 are correct.
b) 1 only is correct.
c) 1, 3 and 4 are correct.
d) all of the above are correct.

16. Examination of Mr. Smith shows dullness and decreased tactile fremitus at the right lung base. You might consider that he has developed a
a) right lower lobe pneumonia.
b) pulmonary edema.
c) right pneumothorax.
d) pleural effusion.

17. Miss Johnson is diagnosed as having a left closed or tension pneumothorax (air in the pleural cavity is open to the bronchi). You would expect to observe
    1. symmetrical lateral lung expansion.
    2. asymmetrical lateral lung expansion.
    3. tracheal deviation to the left.
    4. tracheal deviation to the right.
a) 1 only is correct.
b) 2 and 3 are correct.
c) 1 and 3 are correct.
d) 2 and 4 are correct.
e) none of the above are correct.

18. Mr. Brown has a pneumonia. You note a change in percussion from resonant to dull with an increase in tactile fremitus over the right middle lobe. Therefore you realize that he
a) is improving.
b) is developing an area of consolidation.
c) has pneumothorax.
d) has some atelectasis.

19. A client with emphysema will demonstrate_______________diaphragmatic excursion than (as) normal.
a) greater
b) less
c) the same amount of

20. Air trapped in the pleural space will percuss_______________and demonstrate

_______________tactile fremitus.
    1. dull
    2. hyperresonant
    3. resonant
    4. increased
    5. decreased
a) 1 and 5 are correct.
b) 2 and 4 are correct.
c) 2 and 5 are correct.
d) 3 and 4 are correct.
e) 3 and 5 are correct.

Number 14

Examination of the Respiratory System—Inspection, Palpation, Percussion

RATIONALE

The focus of this self-instructional unit is inspection, palpation and percussion of the thorax. Its purpose is to describe and discuss thoracic configuration, respiratory patterns and rates, topography of lung lobes and examination techniques. At the end of this unit you will be able to complete a general inspection for respiratory function and assess the thorax for configuration, respiratory rate and pattern; palpate for symmetrical expansion, pain or discomfort, tracheal position and tactile fremitus; and finally percuss the thorax, recognizing the patterns of resonance and diaphragmatic excursion.

GLOSSARY OF TERMS

Review these terms before and after completing this unit. You should be able to define or describe them readily.

Angle of Louis (sternal angle) ____

Biot's respirations ____

Bradypnea ____

COPD (chronic obstructive pulmonary
    disease) ____

Cheyne-Stokes respirations ____

Dyspnea ____

Hyperresonance ____

Hyperpnea ____

Kyphosis ____

Kussmaul respirations ____

Orthopnea ____

Pectus carinatum (pigeon breast) ______________________________________

Pectus excavatum (funnel breast) ______________________________________

Pleximeter ____

Resonance ____

Scoliosis ____

Tactile fremitus ____

Tympany ____

COGNITIVE OBJECTIVES

At the end of this unit you will demonstrate knowledge of inspection, palpation and percussion of the respiratory system by your ability to:

1. Systematically list the elements included in inspection of the respiratory system.

2. Correctly locate or diagram the following structures on an anterior, lateral or posterior view of the thorax; angle of Louis, specific ribs or intercostal spaces, spinal segments, borders of the major lobes and fissures of the lungs, xiphoid process, suprasternal notch.

3. List and describe four common thoracic deformities.

4. Describe the following respiratory rates and patterns: normal adult, tachypnea, bradypnea, Cheyne-Stokes, Biot's, Kussmaul.

5. Systematically list the elements included in palpation of the respiratory system.

6. List and describe conditions which cause tracheal deviation.

7. Describe the techniques for palpating expansion of the thorax and identify
   a. one condition which increases expansion.
   b. four conditions which limit lung expansion.
   c. two conditions which result in asymmetrical expansion.

8. Define and describe the procedure for eliciting tactile fremitus.
   a. Identify and describe conditions which interfere with the transmission of sound vibrations.
   b. Identify and describe conditions which favor transmission of vibrations.

9. State a rationale for palpating for tenderness of the spine and costovertebral angle.

10. Systematically list the elements included in percussion during the respiratory examination.

11. Differentiate between the characteristics of tympanic, resonant, dull and flat percussion notes; state conditions in which the percussion note of the lung is altered.

12. List in sequence the steps for determining diaphragmatic excursion; describe four causative factors which can alter excursion.

LEARNING ACTIVITIES

The Learning Activities contain the information necessary for meeting the Cognitive Objectives. Select one and proceed to work with it until you have mastered the material. Use the Cognitive Objectives as a study guide. A Self-Test is provided so that you can check how much you know. If you have difficulty with the Self-Test, please review the material in the unit.

Reading Activities

a) Bates: *A Guide to Physical Examination*, "The Thorax and Lungs." This is a good review of the anatomy and landmarks of the thorax. Inspection, palpation and percussion of the thorax are systematically outlined, with descriptions of normal and abnormal findings. The student will need to do additional reading on respiratory patterns and conditions which increase, limit or result in asymmetrical lung expansion.

b) Delp and Manning: *Major's Physical Diagnosis*, "The Chest, Lungs and Pulmonary System." Anatomical topography of the thorax is reviewed and illustrated. Inspection is somewhat superficially covered, although thoracic deformities and respiratory patterns are well described. Palpation and percussion techniques are presented in detail and related to normal and abnormal findings.

c) DeGowin and DeGowin: *Bedside Diagnostic Examination*, Chapter 6. This reading is divided into inspection and palpation of the thoracic cage and palpation and percussion of the lungs. A review of the anatomy and landmarks is presented with each section. The information for meeting the Cognitive Objectives is presented in this reading, although the student may be overwhelmed by the detail and the number of abnormalities presented.

d) Gillies and Alyn: *Patient Assessment and Management by the Nurse Practitioner*, Chapter 3. This chapter reviews the accepted landmarks of the thorax; additional reading will be necessary to relate lung lobes to ribs and spinous processes. Inspection, palpation and percussion techniques are well outlined with normal findings fully described. Abnormalities are correlated to signs and symptoms.

e) Judge and Zuidema: *Methods of Clinical Examination: A Physiologic Approach*, "The Respiratory System." Anatomy of thorax is demonstrated through a series of drawings and chest x-rays. Inspection, palpation and percussion techniques are discussed in relation to normal findings. Abnormal findings are related to underlying pathophysiology. The approach is systematic and easy to follow.

f) Prior and Silberstein: *Physical Diagnosis*, "Thorax and Lungs." Topography and thoracic landmarks are clearly illustrated and simply explained. The presentation on inspection, palpation and percussion is thorough and also well illustrated. Photographs of examination techniques and normal findings facilitate understanding of the material.

g) Sana and Judge: *Physical Appraisal Methods in Nursing Practice*, "Physical Appraisal of Respiratory System Function." A complete discussion of inspection, palpation and percussion of the thorax and lungs is presented in this chapter. Topography and thoracic landmarks are described and illustrated. Normal and abnormal findings are outlined.

h) Sherman and Fields: *Guide to Patient Evaluation*, "The Thorax and Lungs." This chapter provides a good introductory reading to evaluation of the thorax and lungs. However, additional reading will be necessary to meet the Cognitive Objectives.

Audiovisual Activities

a) Blue-Hill Educational Systems, Inc.: "The Respiratory System," Tape XIA. This 30-minute video tape lecture includes a discussion of thoracic landmarks, inspection of the chest and abnormalities of the thorax and respiratory patterns. Tactile fremitus and percussion of the thorax are covered in depth. The student should refer to a textbook for anatomical relationships between the lung lobes and external landmarks.

b) Concept Media: "Physical Assessment: Heart and Lungs." This filmstrip and audiocassette presentation is designed to introduce you to concepts and skills of physical assessment of the thorax. Program I focuses on inspection and palpation of the lungs and thorax. Programs II and III focus on percussion and auscultation of the lungs.

c) Thiokol-Humetrics: *The Chest: Its Signs and Sounds*. An audiotape presentation with an accompanying book. The first four audiotapes in this series cover the essentials of inspection, palpation and percussion of the chest. Helpful for the beginning practitioner are the frequent examples of sounds heard on percussion.

d) Westinghouse Learning Health Services: "Examination of the Thorax and Lungs." This self-instructional package consists of filmstrips, audiocassettes and student workbooks. Focus is on evaluating thoracic configuration, respiratory patterns and percussion notes.

SELF-TEST

This Self-Test is for you. Use it to check how well you have learned the material in this unit. The answers follow the test.

1. Inspection of the respiratory system includes assessment of
   1. movement of the diaphragm.
   2. respiratory rate, depth and rhythm.
   3. symmetry of chest excursion.
   4. fremitus.
   5. skeletal or postural deformity.
   a) 2 and 5 are correct.
   b) 1, 2, 3 and 5 are correct.
   c) 1, 2, 4 and 5 are correct.
   d) 2, 3 and 5 are correct.
   e) all of the above are correct.

2. Name the structures or anatomical landmarks labeled in the accompanying drawing.

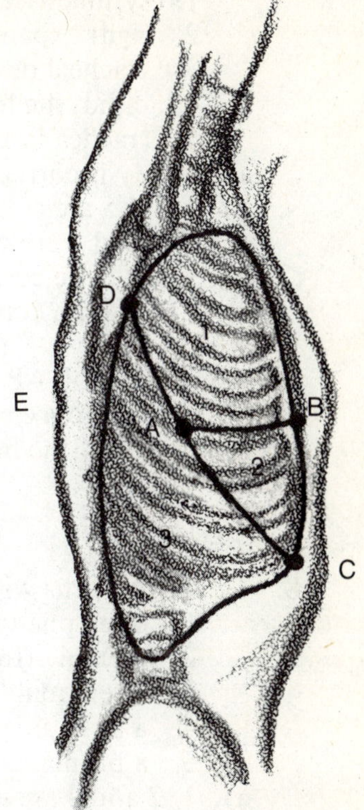

1) _______________ lobe

2) _______________ lobe

3) _______________ lobe

A) _______________ rib (midaxillary line)

B) _______________ rib (midclavicular line)

C) _______________ rib (midclavicular line)

D) _______________ spinous process

E) _______________ fissure

3. Draw a lateral view of the spine showing the cervical, thoracic and lumbar curvatures found in kyphosis.

4. Regular, very deep respirations seen in diabetic acidosis are called _______________ respirations.
    a) bradypneic
    b) Kussmaul's
    c) Biot's
    d) Cheyne-Stokes

5. Palpation of the respiratory system does *not* include assessment of
    a) tactile fremitus.
    b) chest expansion.
    c) evidence of masses or tumors.
    d) tracheal position.
    e) depth of respiration.

6. Ms. Clarke's diagnosis is right open pneumothorax. You would expect to find
   1. symmetrical lung expansion.
   2. right expansion greater than left.
   3. tracheal deviation to the right.
   4. rapid, shallow breathing and cyanosis.
   5. trachea in the midline.
   a) 4 only is correct.
   b) 1 and 5 are correct.
   c) 2, 3 and 4 are correct.
   d) 2 and 5 are correct.
   e) 1 and 4 are correct.

7. Assessment of AP diameter can be made by placing one hand on each side of the posterior thorax, asking the client to inhale deeply and noting symmetry of movement of the hands.
   a) True
   b) False

8. Tactile fremitus will be decreased with
   1. open pneumothorax.
   2. pleural effusion.
   3. pneumonia.
   4. a large area of atelectasis.
   5. a bronchial plug.
   a) 1, 2 and 4 are correct.
   b) 3 only is correct.
   c) 1, 2, 4 and 5 are correct.
   d) none of the above are correct.
   e) all of the above are correct.

9. Assessment of the respiratory system by percussion includes
   1. comparison of symmetrical areas of both lung fields.
   2. location of the bases of the lungs during inspiration and expiration.
   3. perception of the character of vibrations that can be heard as well as felt.
   4. placing the pleximeter horizontally over the rib, not the interspace.
   5. perception of relative densities.
   a) 1, 3 and 4 are correct.
   b) 3 and 5 are correct.
   c) 2 and 4 are correct.
   d) 1, 2, 3 and 5 are correct.
   e) all of the above are correct.

10. An increased volume of air in the lung will create a _______________ percussion note.
    a) flat
    b) resonant
    c) dull
    d) hyperresonant
    e) none of the above

11. Movement of the diaphragm is decreased by
    1. COPD.
    2. pregnancy.
    3. paralysis of the phrenic nerve.

    4. positive pressure in the thorax.
    5. a large abdominal mass.
a) 2, 3 and 5 are correct.
b) 1 and 4 are correct.
c) 5 only is correct.
d) none of the above are correct.
e) all of the above are correct.

12. Which of the following is not usually a sign of respiratory dysfunction?
    a) continuous, sharp chest pain
    b) cyanosis
    c) sternal retraction
    d) productive cough
    e) clubbing of digits

SELF-TEST KEY

1. (d) Abnormal respiratory rate, depth or rhythm; unequal movement of the sides of the chest; or deformity can indicate dysfunction. Diaphragmatic excursion is rarely observed accurately and is better determined by percussion. Fremitus is not visible.

2. (1) right upper lobe
    (2) right middle lobe
    (3) right lower lobe
    (A) 5th rib (midaxillary line)
    (B) 4th rib (midclavicular line)
    (C) 6th rib (midclavicular line)
    (D) T2 or T3 spinous process
    (E) Oblique fissure

3. Kyphosis is a skeletal abnormality which demonstrates an exaggerated posterior curvature of the thoracic spine. The cervical and lumbar spines are relatively normal anterior curves.

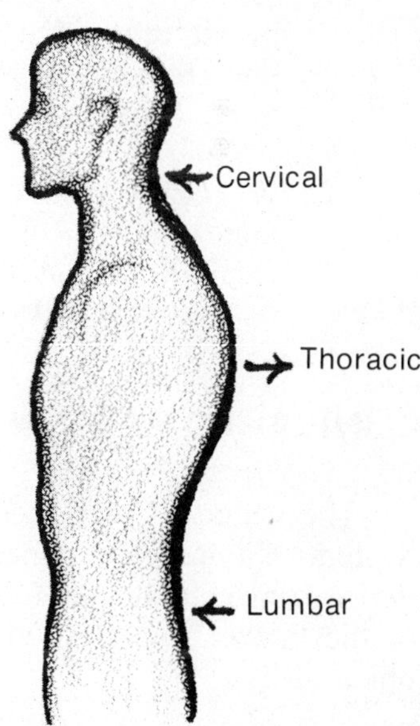

4. (b) Kussmaul's respirations. Bradypneic respiration is slow, regular breathing associated with drug overdose and coma. Biot's respiration is a form of cyclical breathing, alternating apnea with periods of breaths of equal depth which end suddenly. Cheyne-Stokes respiration is cyclical breathing which is marked by periods

of apnea, slow shallow respirations, rapid deep respirations, slow shallow respirations and then apnea.

5. (e) Abnormalities of transmission of air vibrations through the chest wall or AP and lateral chest expansion, areas tender to palpation and deviation of the trachea are palpable signs of respiratory dysfunction. Depth of respiration is generally included under inspection.

6. (a) With a right open pneumothorax, the pressure in the right thoracic cavity increases to atmospheric pressure, collapsing the entire lung: the mediastinal contents are pulled to the left by the normal negative pressure. The client shows signs of respiratory distress.

7. (b) This is the procedure for evaluating lateral expansion.

8. (c) Tactile fremitus is diminished when airways are blocked or air or fluid in the pleural space damps transmission of voice vibrations. Pneumonia increases the density of lung tissue open to the bronchi and facilitates transmission of vibrations.

9. (d) Percussion includes assessing symmetrical areas of both lung fields, diaphragmatic excursion, and hearing and feeling vibrations produced by striking over structures of differing densities. Percussion over a rib would distort the findings.

10. (d) Hyperresonant. Hyperinflation of the alveoli increases the normal resonance. Flatness is percussed over bone; dullness is percussed over a dense organ such as the heart or liver; tympany is percussed over a hollow structure such as an empty stomach.

11. (e) A lowered diaphragm may be caused by increased air in the lung as in COPD or by air or fluid in the pleural space. A raised diaphragm occurs with injury to the phrenic nerve or a large space-occupying abdominal mass such as a tumor, pregnancy or ascites.

12. (a) Chest pain of respiratory origin is generally related to the respiratory cycle, increasing or decreasing with respirations. Chest pain which is unaffected by respirations may be cardiac in origin or may be pain referred from abdominal viscera.

CLINICAL COMPONENT

The Clinical Component for Units 14 and 15 is presented in Unit 16, The Respiratory System: Clinical Component (p. 279). Preview the Clinical Objectives in that unit and the Performance Guide cards for Unit 16 in Appendix II for inspection, palpation and percussion of the thorax. Facilitate your learning by practicing these skills before proceeding to the next unit.

Name_______________________________

Date_______________________________

PRE-TEST

UNIT 15

Choose the *one* best answer.

1. Wheezes are
   1. heard better on expiration.
   2. heard better on inspiration.
   3. associated with diffusion defects.
   4. associated with narrowing of airways.
   a) 1 and 3 are correct.
   b) 2 and 3 are correct.
   c) 1 and 4 are correct.
   d) 4 only is correct.

2. Vesicular breath sounds
   1. are heard over most of the thorax.
   2. are due to distention of alveoli during inspiration.
   3. have an inspiratory component that is more intense, higher pitched and longer in duration than the expiratory component.
   4. have approximately equal inspiratory and expiratory phases.
   a) 1, 2 and 3 are correct.
   b) 1, 2 and 4 are correct.
   c) 2 and 4 are correct.
   d) 1 and 2 are correct.

3. Obesity, pneumonectomy and pleural effusions cause
   1. increased breath sounds.
   2. decreased or absent breath sounds.
   3. asthmatic breath sounds.
   4. cavernous breath sounds.
   a) 1 and 3 are correct.
   b) 2 only is correct.
   c) 1 and 4 are correct.
   d) 4 only is correct.

4. Bronchial breath sounds are normal if heard
   a) between the scapulae.
   b) over the trachea.
   c) over the manubrium.
   d) over the clavicles.

5. Inflamed, roughened pleural layers produce
   a) gurgling rales.
   b) rhonchi.
   c) wheezes.
   d) rubs.

6. Asthmatic breath sounds produce an expiratory phase that is
   a) markedly long.
   b) markedly short.

7. Examine the following diagrams of breath sounds. Which one represents a bronchovesicular breath sound?

   a)   b)   c)   d)

8. Low-pitched, discrete sounds with a bubbling quality produced by air passing through fluid in the larger airways are called
   a) rales.
   b) rhonchi.
   c) rubs.
   d) wheezes.

9. Fine, moist, high-pitched crackling sounds are
   a) rales.
   b) rhonchi.
   c) rubs.
   d) wheezes.

10. Rales are usually heard on
    a) inspiration.
    b) expiration.

11. Breath sounds which are muffled, blowing and have approximately equal inspiration and expiration phases are
    a) vesicular.
    b) bronchial.
    c) bronchovesicular.
    d) tracheal.

12. Bronchovesicular breath sounds are normally auscultated
    a) at the base of the lungs.
    b) between the scapulae.

13. Breath sounds are absent in
    1. pneumothorax.
    2. pneumonia.
    3. complete airway obstruction.
    4. COPD
    a) 1 only is correct.
    b) 1, 2 and 3 are correct.
    c) 1 and 3 are correct.
    d) all of the above are correct.

14. Rhonchi can be caused by
    1. mucus plugs.
    2. tumor growth.
    3. bronchitis.
    4. food aspiration.

    a) 1 and 3 are correct.
    b) 1, 2 and 3 are correct.
    c) 1 only is correct.
    d) all of the above are correct.

15. Fine rales
      1. disappear with coughing.
      2. move with positioning.
      3. are heard at the end of inspiration.
      4. are due to bronchoconstriction.
    a) all of the above are correct.
    b) 1 and 3 are correct.
    c) 1, 2 and 3 are correct.
    d) 1 only is correct.

16. Auscultatory examination of your client reveals diminished vesicular breath sounds. This could be due to
      1. obesity.
      2. emphysema.
      3. a thickened pleural lining.
      4. pulmonary consolidation.
    a) 1 only is correct.
    b) 1, 2 and 3 are correct.
    c) 4 only is correct.
    d) all of the above are correct.

17. Your client has a massive pneumonia. You would expect to hear
      1. vesicular breath sounds.
      2. coarse rales or rhonchi.
      3. E to A change with vocal fremitus.
      4. increased transmission of whispered words.
    a) 1 and 2 are correct.
    b) 4 only is correct.
    c) 2, 3 and 4 are correct.
    d) all of the above are correct.

18. In COPD in which there is overinflation and destruction of the alveoli, breath sounds will be
    a) increased.
    b) decreased.
    c) normal.

19. Mr. Smith complains of wheezing. This could be due to
      1. mucus-plugged bronchi.
      2. mucosal swelling of airways.
      3. airways narrowed with secretions.
      4. friction from an inflamed pleura.
    a) 3 only is correct.
    b) 1 and 2 are correct.
    c) 2 and 3 are correct.
    d) all of the above are correct.

20. While auscultating Ms. Brown's lungs you note vesicular breath sounds in the left lower lobe and bronchovesicular sounds in the right middle lobe. You suspect that she has
    a) pleural disease on the left.
    b) localized obstructive lung disease.
    c) an area of developing consolidation.
    d) a right middle lobe pneumothorax.

Number 15

Examination of the Respiratory System—Auscultation

RATIONALE

The focus of this self-instructional unit is auscultation of the lungs. Its purpose is to introduce you to lung sounds. At the end of this unit you will be able to systematically assess respiratory functions: identify breath sounds which are considered normal for the underlying lung tissue; verbally describe the characteristics of abnormal and adventitious breath sounds, and correlate them with conditions in which they would be found.

GLOSSARY OF TERMS

Review the following terms before and after completing this unit. You should be able to define or describe them readily.

Asthma ____

Atelectasis ____

Bronchitis ____

Bronchophony ____

Bronchovesicular ____

Egophony ____

Emphysema ____

Friction rub ____

Pectoriloquy ____

Rales ____

Rhonchi ____

Vesicular ____

Wheeze ____

COGNITIVE OBJECTIVES

At the end of this unit you will demonstrate knowledge of auscultation of the respiratory system by your ability to:

1. Describe and diagram the inspiratory and expiratory phases which differentiate vesicular, bronchovesicular and bronchial (tracheal) breath sounds.

2. Outline the areas in which vesicular, bronchovesicular and bronchial breath sounds are normally auscultated, on a diagram on the anterior and posterior thorax.

3. Identify conditions in which bronchovesicular and bronchial breath sounds would be considered abnormal.

4. List five conditions in which breath sounds are decreased or absent.

5. Differentiate rales, rhonchi, wheezes and pleural rubs in relation to anatomical location, intensity and time in the respiratory cycle.

6. Identify the pathophysiological basis for development of rales, rhonchi, wheezes and pleural rubs.

7. Recognize the characteristics of breath sounds which commonly occur in the following respiratory conditions:
   a. Pneumonia
   b. Pneumothorax
   c. COPD
   d. Asthma
   e. Bronchitis
   f. Pleurisy

8. Define bronchophony, egophony and whispered pectoriloquy.

LEARNING ACTIVITIES

The Learning Activities contain the information necessary for meeting the Cognitive Objectives. Select one and proceed to work with it until you have mastered the material. Use the Cognitive Objectives as a study guide. A Self-Test is provided so that you can check how much you know. If you have difficulty with the Self-Test, please review the material in this unit.

Reading Activities

a) Bates: *A Guide to Physical Examination*, "The Thorax and Lungs." Breath sounds are not diagrammed, but their duration, pitch and location are fully described. Abnormal and adventitious breath sounds are described and related to common respiratory conditions in the table at the end of the chapter.

b) Delp and Manning: *Major's Physical Diagnosis*, "Examination of Chest, Lungs and Pulmonary System," pp. 334–351. Vesicular and bronchial breath sounds are well described. The authors have chosen to omit bronchovesicular sounds. Abnormal and adventitious sounds are related to underlying pathology, anatomical origin, intensity and time in the respiratory cycle. The format of this presentation mandates careful reading by the beginning student.

c) DeGowin and DeGowin: *Bedside Diagnostic Examination*, "The Lungs and Pleura," pp. 295–314. The information needed to meet the objectives is well presented in this chapter. The emphasis on differential diagnosis may confuse the beginning practitioner; other readings are recommended.

d) Gillies and Alyn: *Patient Assessment and Management by the Nurse Practitioner*, "Auscultation," pp. 75–78. Complete information for meeting the Cognitive Objectives is not contained in this reading. However, the discussion on normal and adventitious breath sounds is clear and concise and provides a good introduction to auscultation.

e) Judge and Zuidema: *Methods of Clinical Examination: A Physiologic Approach*, "Respiratory System." Normal breath sounds and auscultatory techniques are clearly described. The discussion on abnormal and adventitious breath sounds is descriptive; application is to pathophysiological phenomena rather than to specific disease entities.

f) Prior and Silberstein: *Physical Diagnosis*, "Thorax and Lungs," pp. 192–200. Breath sounds are analyzed and diagrammed. Abnormal breath sounds and voice sounds are clearly described and related to common conditions. The discussion on adventitious breath sounds is simple and concise. This reading is well illustrated, and the presentation has an easy flow.

g) Sana and Judge: *Physical Appraisal Methods in Nursing Practice*, "Physical Appraisal of Respiratory System Function." A clear, well-illustrated discussion of normal, abnormal and adventitious breath sounds and voice sounds. Examination techniques and normal variants are also outlined in this reading.

h) Sherman and Fields: *Guide to Patient Evaluation*, "The Thorax and Lung." This reading presents an adequate overview of auscultation techniques and breath sounds. Salient information is presented but not fully described or related to underlying pathophysiological conditions. Students may find the example for recording findings at the end of this chapter very helpful.

Audiovisual Activities

a) Blue-Hill Educational Systems, Inc.: "Respiratory – Part XIB." This video tape program includes discussions of the stethoscope and normal, abnormal and adventitious breath sounds. The lecture concludes with a demonstration of the thoracic examination.

b) Concept Media: "Physical Assessment: Heart and Lungs." This filmstrip and audiotape presentation is designed to introduce the student to the concepts and skills of physical assessment of the thorax. Auscultation is presented along with percussion in programs II and III of this series.

c) Thiokol-Humetrics: "The Chest: Its Signs and Sounds." This is an audiotape presentation with accompanying text. Tapes 5 through 8 describe proper use of the stethoscope and normal, abnormal and adventitious breath sounds. Content is presented clearly and concisely; breath sounds are demonstrated throughout.

d) Westinghouse Learning Health Service: "Examination of the Thorax and Lungs." In this filmstrip/audiocassette tape program developed by Sherman and Fields, emphasis is on differentiating breath sounds and recognizing abnormal and adventitious breath sounds and voice sounds. Recording methodology is also included in the program series.

SELF-TEST

This Self-Test is for you. Use it to check how well you have learned the material presented in the unit. The answers to the questions follow the test.

1. Diagram the inspiratory and expiratory phases of vesicular, bronchovesicular, bronchial and asthmatic breath sounds.

2. On the accompanying illustration, label and draw the locations where *normal* breath sounds are heard, using the following symbols:
   /// vesicular
   x bronchovesicular
   o bronchial

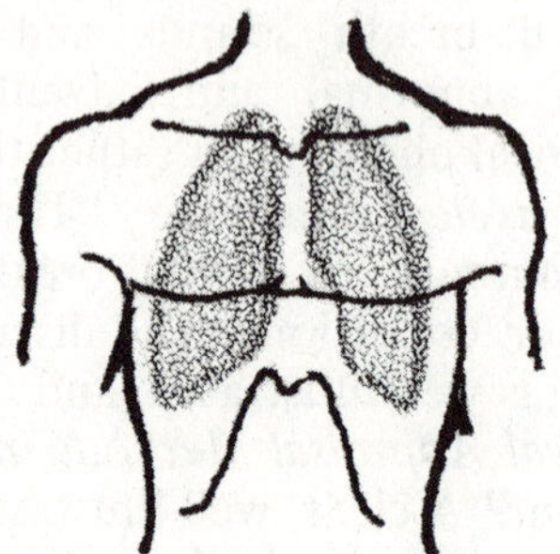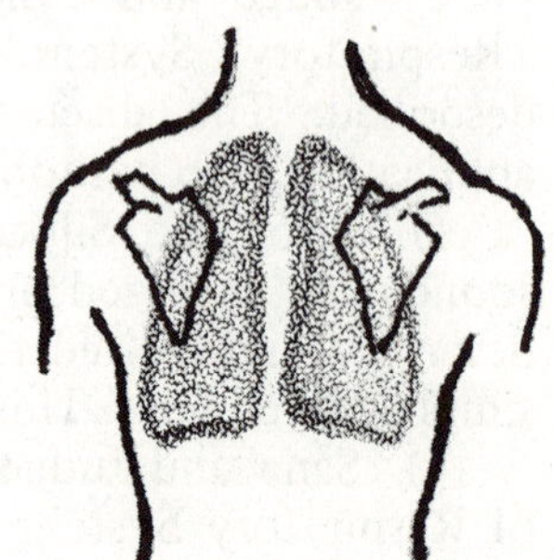

3. Bronchovesicular or bronchial breath sounds are heard in the lower lung field. This may indicate
   1. a normal variation.
   2. consolidation.
   3. compressed lung tissue.
   4. hyperinflation of alveoli.
   5. a bronchial plug.
   a) 2, 3 and 5 are correct.
   b) 4 only is correct.
   c) 3 and 5 are correct.
   d) 1 only is correct.
   e) 2 and 3 are correct.

4. Diminished or absent breath sounds occur in
   1. emphysema.
   2. bronchial plug.
   3. obesity.
   4. pneumothorax.
   5. a small pleural effusion.
   a) 2 only is correct.
   b) 1 and 3 are correct.
   c) 4 and 5 are correct.
   d) 1, 2, 3 and 4 are correct.
   e) all of the above are correct.

5. Rhonchi are
   1. low-pitched, loud, gurgling sounds.
   2. heard only on inspiration.

    3. high-pitched, crackling sounds.
    4. produced by passage of air through fluid in the larger airways.
    5. frequently heard in atelectasis.
a) 1, 2, 4 and 5 are correct.
b) 1 and 4 are correct.
c) 2 and 3 are correct.
d) 2 and 4 are correct.
e) 3 and 5 are correct.

6. Pleural friction rubs
    1. are heard on inspiration and expiration.
    2. are caused by fluid in the pleura.
    3. disappear with coughing.
    4. are characteristically high-pitched, fizzy and musical.
    5. are frequently transient.
a) 1, 2, 3 and 4 are correct.
b) 2, 4 and 5 are correct.
c) 1 and 5 are correct.
d) all of the above are correct.
e) none of the above are correct.

7. Ms. Marble has bronchitis. You might expect to find
    1. inspiratory stridor.
    2. a pleural friction rub.
    3. wheezes, rales or rhonchi.
    4. bronchophony.
    5. normal or prolonged expiration.
a) 1, 3 and 4 are correct.
b) 3 only is correct.
c) 3 and 5 are correct.
d) 2, 4 and 5 are correct.
e) all of the above are correct.

SELF-TEST KEY

1. Vesicular: long inspiratory, short expiratory
    Bronchovesicular: inspiratory and expiratory phases approximately
      equal
    Bronchial: short inspiratory, long expiratory
    Asthmatic: short inspiratory; very long, high-pitched expiratory due
      to narrowing of airways during expiration

2. Vesicular breath sounds are heard over the entire lung field.
    Bronchovesicular breath sounds are heard over the manubrium and upper intrascapular areas.
    Bronchial breath sounds are *not* normal breath sounds (simulate by listening over the trachea).

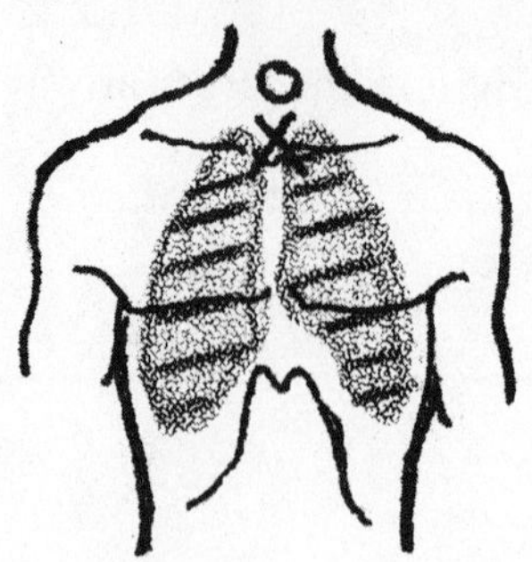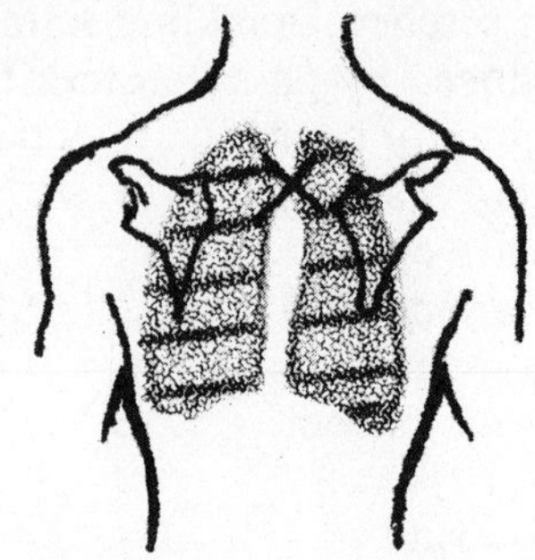

3. (e) Bronchovesicular and bronchial breath sounds in the lung field are always abnormal and are caused by varying degrees of consolidation or compression of pulmonary tissue which facilitates transmission of sound from the bronchi to the chest wall. No sound is transmitted when the airway is blocked.

4. (e) Breath sounds are diminished or absent when the airway is blocked, the distance between the chest wall and lung is increased, sound vibrations are damped by fluid or air in the pleural space or the pleura is thickened.

5. (b) Rhonchi (or coarse rales) are caused by movement of air through fluid or exudate in the larger airways. They have a loud, low-pitched, gurgling quality and are more prominent during expiration. Atelectasis is the collapse of alveoli.

6. (c) Friction rubs are coarse, grating sounds caused by pleural surfaces rubbing together when there is a lack of lubricating fluid or inflammation. The rub is heard on inspiration and expiration, is unaffected by coughing (rales usually are) and is generally transient because of intermittent lubrication.

7. (c) In bronchitis, abnormalities are due to bronchial secretions which cause adventitious sounds and may increase expiration time if air is trapped in alveoli by secretions. The pleura and lung tissue are not affected.

CLINICAL COMPONENT

The Clinical Component for Units 14 and 15 is presented in Unit 16, The Respiratory System: Clinical Component. Preview the Clinical Objectives in that unit and the Performance Guide cards for Unit 16 in Appendix II for auscultation of the lungs.

Number 16

The Respiratory System: Clinical Component

You are now ready to proceed to the Clinical Objectives for examination of the respiratory system. The purpose of the clinical component is to help you practice assessment of respiratory function and learn detection of the presence, location and extent of any dysfunction.

CLINICAL OBJECTIVES

At the end of this unit you will be able to perform an assessment of the respiratory system, correlating physical examination skills and physiological principles. You will:

1. Demonstrate knowledge of signs and symptoms of respiratory dysfunction by obtaining a pertinent health history.

2. Demonstrate inspection of the thorax by systematically assessing general body build, skin color, nail beds, thoracic configuration, rate and pattern of respirations and movement of the thorax.

3. Demonstrate palpation of the thorax by
   a. estimating AP and lateral chest expansion.
   b. locating any areas of tenderness.
   c. identifying the position of the trachea.
   d. systematically comparing tactile fremitus in symmetrical areas of the chest.

4. Demonstrate indirect percussion of the thorax by eliciting percussion notes in various lobes of the lung.

5. Demonstrate the technique for determining diaphragmatic excursion by percussion.

6. Demonstrate systematic auscultation of the lung by
   a. identifying the characteristics of normal, abnormal and adventitious breath sounds in each lobe and comparing for symmetry.
   b. checking abnormal findings by tests for bronchophony, egophony and whispered pectoriloquy.

7. Utilize S.O.A.P. to systematically describe your findings, make an assessment of respiratory function and formulate a plan of action.

INSTRUCTIONS

Utilizing three of your peers or clients in the clinical area, practice inspection, palpation, percussion and auscultation of the thorax and lungs. Remove the Performance Guide cards for Unit 16 from Appendix II. These cards will enable you to practice the skills necessary to meet the Clinical Objectives and complete the Response Sheets. On each Response Sheet you will be expected to (1) ask questions which elicit possible symptoms, (2) systematically describe your findings, (3) localize any abnormalities present and (4) summarize your examination findings using the S.O.A.P. method of recording.

When you have mastered the Clinical Objectives and completed the Response Sheets, arrange to demonstrate your skills to your laboratory instructor or preceptor.

EQUIPMENT

Stethoscope

OPTIONAL ACTIVITIES

These activities demonstrate techniques for assessment of the respiratory system.

a) Bates: "The Thorax." This film demonstrates thoracic examination procedures.

b) Blue-Hill Educational Systems, Inc.: "Respiratory Examination." This video tape cassette presentation concerns techniques of respiratory physical assessment.

Client ________________________________

Date ____________________ Age ________ Sex ________

Examiner ______________________________

I. Health History

II. Physical Examination

A. Inspection

   1. General

   2. Chest configuration

   3. Respiratory rate

   4. Respiratory pattern

B. Palpation

   1. Lateral and AP chest expansion

   2. Tenderness

   3. Trachea

    4. Tactile fremitus

C. Percussion

    1. Resonance

    2. Diaphragmatic excursion

D. Auscultation

    1. Breath sounds

    2. Abnormal breath sounds

    3. Adventitious sounds

Summarize your findings using the S.O.A.P. method.

S.   (Client's observations, complaints, health history)

O.   (Physical findings)
Diagram your findings on the accompanying drawing.

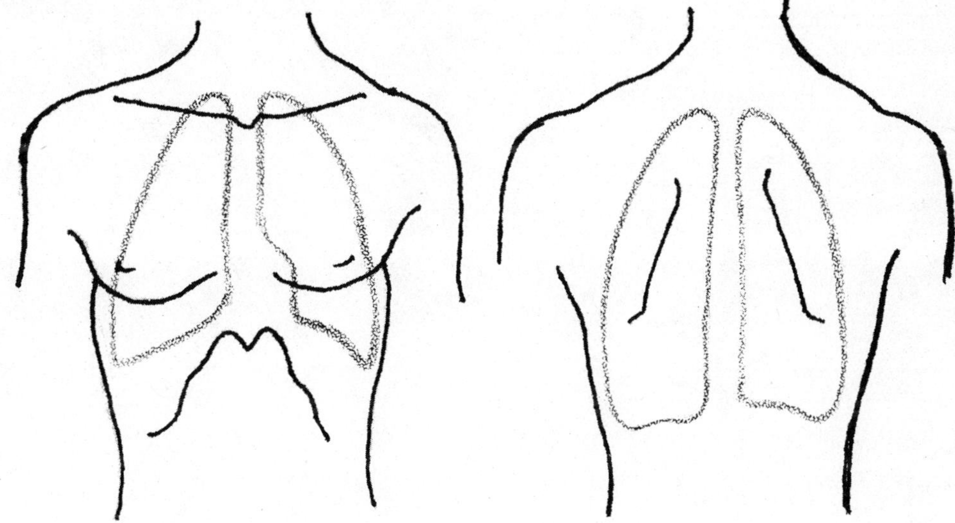

A.   (Assessment of problem, data, prognosis)

P.   (Plans for further evaluation, care, teaching)

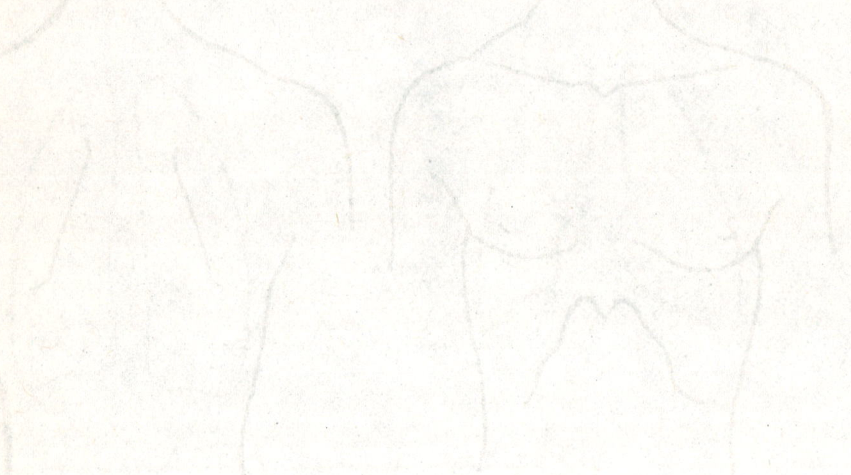

RESPONSE SHEET—THE RESPIRATORY SYSTEM

Client _______________________________

Date _______________ Age _______ Sex _____

Examiner _______________________________

I. Health History

II. Physical Examination

A. Inspection

1. General

2. Chest configuration

3. Respiratory rate

4. Respiratory pattern

B. Palpation

1. Lateral and AP chest expansion

2. Tenderness

3. Trachea

4. Tactile fremitus

C. Percussion

1. Resonance

2. Diaphragmatic excursion

D. Auscultation

1. Breath sounds

2. Abnormal breath sounds

3. Adventitious sounds

Summarize your findings using the S.O.A.P. method.

S.   (Client's observations, complaints, health history)

O.   (Physical findings)
Diagram your findings on the accompanying drawing.

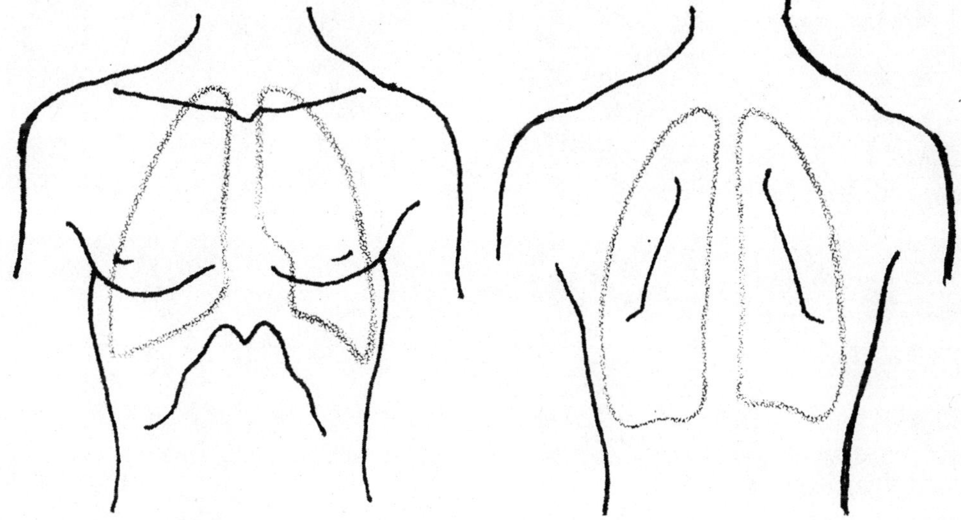

A.   (Assessment of problem, data, prognosis)

P.   (Plans for further evaluation, care, teaching)

Client _______________________________

Date _________________ Age _______ Sex _______

Examiner _____________________________

I. Health History

II. Physical Examination

A. Inspection

1. General

2. Chest configuration

3. Respiratory rate

4. Respiratory pattern

B. Palpation

1. Lateral and AP chest expansion

2. Tenderness

3. Trachea

4. Tactile fremitus

C. Percussion

1. Resonance

2. Diaphragmatic excursion

D. Auscultation

1. Breath sounds

2. Abnormal breath sounds

3. Adventitious sounds

Summarize your findings using the S.O.A.P. method.

S. **(Client's observations, complaints, health history)**

O. **(Physical findings)**
Diagram your findings on the accompanying drawing.

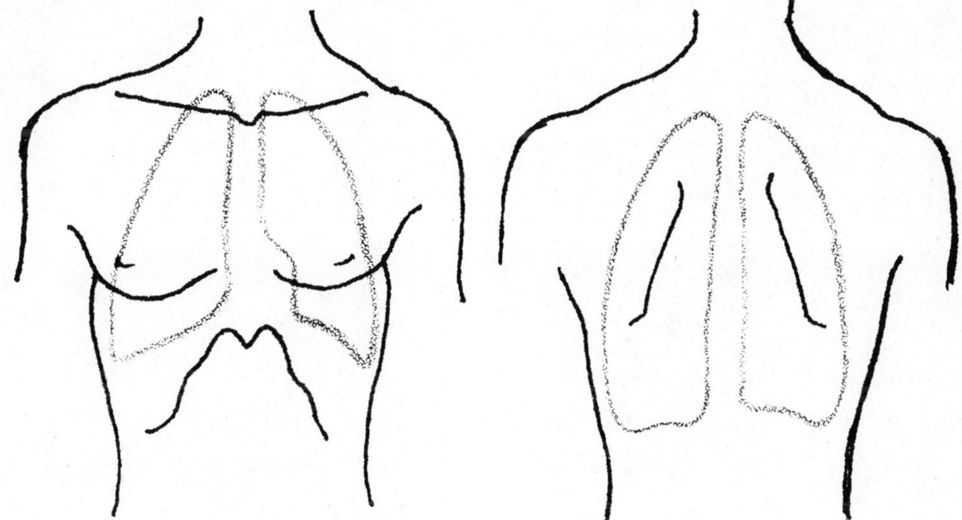

A. **(Assessment of problem, data, prognosis)**

P. **(Plans for further evaluation, care, teaching)**

PRE-TEST

UNIT 17

1. Precordial inspection includes
   1. configuration of the thorax.
   2. chest wall pulsations.
   3. observation for dyspnea and tachypnea.
   4. neck vein distention.
   5. clubbing of the fingers.
   a) 1, 2 and 4 are correct.
   b) 1, 2 and 3 are correct.
   c) 2, 4 and 5 are correct.
   d) all of the above are correct.

Locate the following structures on the accompanying diagram.

2. _______ Pulmonary arteries

3. _______ Apex

4. _______ Aorta

5. _______ Right ventricle

6. _______ Right atrium

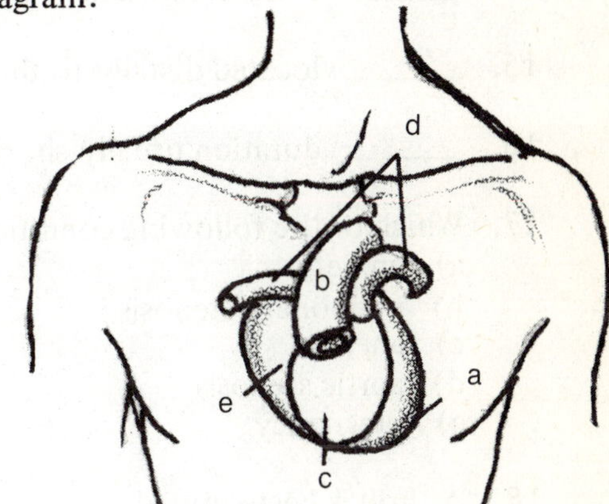

7. The midclavicular line is
   a) a horizontal line between the angle of Louis and the acromioclavicular joint.
   b) a vertical line midway between the midsternal line and acromioclavicular joint.
   c) a perpendicular line from the anterior axillary fold.
   d) a line midway between the anterior axillary fold and midsternal line.

8. The primary area for inspecting and palpating the aortic valve is
   a) in the 2nd intercostal space to the left of the sternum.
   b) in the 4th intercostal space 2–3 cm to the left of the sternum.
   c) in the 2nd intercostal space to the right of the sternum.
   d) in the 3rd intercostal space to the left of the sternum.

9. The tricuspid area is inspected and palpated
   a) just below the xiphoid.
   b) 7–9 cm to the left of the sternum.
   c) immediately over the sternum at the level of the 3rd rib.
   d) in the 5th intercostal space to the immediate left of the sternum and the lower
      left sternal border.

293

10. The part of the hand that is most sensitive to precordial vibrations such as thrills is
    a) the palmar surface.
    b) the ulnar surface.
    c) the fingertips.
    d) none of the above areas.

11. The apex or mitral area of the heart is palpated in the
    a) left 5th intercostal space close to the sternum.
    b) left 5th intercostal space 2–4 cm from the sternum.
    c) left 5th intercostal space 7–9 cm from the sternum.
    d) left 5th intercostal space distal to the midclavicular line.

Identify the following descriptions of the apical impulse as those of the normal apical impulse (A) or left ventricular hypertrophy (B).

12. _______ 3 cm or more in diameter (size)

13. _______ duration lasts throughout systole

14. _______ small amplitude – sometimes absent

15. _______ located distally to the midclavicular line

16. _______ duration usually shorter than one-half of systole

17. Which of the following conditions would *not* produce right ventricular heave?
    a) anxiety
    b) pulmonary stenosis
    c) anemia
    d) aortic stenosis
    e) pregnancy

18. A thrill is best defined as a
    a) palpable cardiac murmur.
    b) retraction of the rib cage.
    c) palpable heart sound.
    d) forceful downward pulsation in the epigastrium.

19. Which of the following would create a pulsation in the aortic area?
    a) aortic stenosis
    b) aortic aneurysm
    c) mitral stenosis
    d) pulmonary hypertension

20. An apical diastolic thrill may be palpable with
    a) aortic stenosis.
    b) patent ductus arteriosus.
    c) tricuspid insufficiency.
    d) severe mitral stenosis.

Number 17

Examination of the Cardiovascular System — Inspection and Palpation

RATIONALE

This self-instructional unit is designed to help you learn inspection and palpation of the precordium. The unit concentrates on thoracic observations and examination of precordial pulsations. At the end of this unit you will be able to demonstrate knowledge of cardiac pulsations by systematically describing the five areas of inspection and palpation and differentiating between normal and abnormal findings.

GLOSSARY OF TERMS

Review the following terms before and after completing this unit. You should be able to define or describe them readily.

Aneurysm ____

Angle of Louis ____

Angina pectoris ____

Apex of the heart ____

Base (cardiac) ____

Clubbing ____

Cor pulmonale ____

Cyanosis ____

Dextrocardia ____

Diastole ____

Dyspnea ____

Edema ____

Erb's point ____

ICS (intercostal space) ____

LVH (left ventricular hypertrophy) _____________________________________

Midclavicular line (MCL)____

Myocardial infarction ____

Orthopnea ____

Palpitation ____

Paroxsymal nocturnal dyspnea (PND)___________________________________

Plethora ____

PMI (point of maximal impulse) ____

Precordium____

Rubs____

Syncope ____

Systole____

Thrill ____

COGNITIVE OBJECTIVES

At the end of this unit you will demonstrate knowledge of inspection and palpation of the precordium by your ability to:

1. Identify the anatomical positions of the right atrium, left atrium, right ventricle, left ventricle, apex of heart, pulmonary artery and aorta on a drawing of the anterior chest.

2. Locate on a drawing the following clinical points of reference:
    a. Midsternal line
    b. Midclavicular line
    c. Anterior axillary line
    d. Midaxillary line

3. Recognize the following clinical areas of inspection and palpation and describe their location on the precordium.
    a. Apical area
    b. Tricuspid area
    c. Erb's point
    d. Pulmonary area
    e. Aortic area
    f. Epigastric area

4. Identify the only pulsation normally observed on the precordium.

5. Define PMI and systematically describe its normal character in relation to
    a. location
    b. duration
    c. amplitude
    d. size

6. Discuss normal variations which may effect the location of the PMI.

7. Compare the characteristics of the normal PMI with the characteristics of the PMI in left ventricular hypertrophy.

8. Identify those cardiac abnormalities which may produce precordial pulsations, thrills or heaves in the
    a. apical area
    b. tricuspid area
    c. aortic area
    d. pulmonary area

LEARNING ACTIVITIES

The Learning Activities each contain the information necessary for meeting the Cognitive Objectives. Select one and proceed to work with it until you have mastered the material. Use the Cognitive Objectives as a study guide. A Self-Test is provided so that you can check how much you know. If you have difficulty with the Self-Test, please review the material in this unit.

Reading Activities

a) Bates: *A Guide to Physical Examination*, "The Heart." This discussion of the anatomy and physiology of the heart is accompanied by several illustrations outlining the dynamics. The student should scan the chapter to locate the pages which discuss the techniques of inspection and palpation of the precordium and the table which lists the abnormalities of apical rates and rhythms.

b) Delp and Manning: *Major's Physical Diagnosis*, "The Cardiovascular System," pp. 358–375. Emphasis in this chapter is predominantly on abnormal findings. The discussion on PMI is very thorough. Several illustrations aid understanding, but additional reading may be necessary.

c) DeGowin and DeGowin: *Bedside Diagnostic Examination*, "The Heart," pp. 326–333. Techniques of inspection and palpation of the precordium are presented. Discussion of PMI is inadequate to meet Cognitive Objectives. Differentiation between normal and abnormal findings is outlined.

d) Gillies and Alyn: *Patient Assessment and Management by the Nurse Practitioner*, "Cardiac Examination," pp. 78–80. Brief overview of the techniques and findings on inspection and palpation of the precordium. Additional readings will be necessary to meet the Cognitive Objectives.

e) Judge and Zuidema: *Methods of Clinical Examination: A Physiologic Approach*. Clinical areas of inspection and palpation are illustrated, and normal findings are discussed. Characteristics of PMI are not well described. Abnormalities are related to underlying physiological mechanisms.

f) Prior and Silberstein: *Physical Diagnosis*, "The Cardiovascular System – The Heart." Discussion relates importance of health history and physical examination to accurate assessment. Anatomical landmarks, inspection, palpation and normal and abnormal findings of precordial pulsations are presented in a concise, readable format.

g) Sana and Judge: *Physical Appraisal Methods in Nursing Practice*, "Physical Appraisal of Circulatory Function." This reading offers a good discussion on examination techniques. Description of normal PMI and PMI in left ventricular hypertrophy is limited. Abnormalities are listed and related to underlying cardiac dysfunction. The student should refer to the respiratory chapter for clinical landmarks and scan the chapter on circulatory function for illustrations of clinical areas of inspection and palpation of the precordium.

h) Sherman and Fields: *Guide to Patient Evaluation*, "The Heart." This chapter provides a basic introduction to the concepts of inspection and palpation of the precordium. Students may wish to utilize this text before moving on to other readings which contain the additional content needed to meet the Cognitive Objectives.

Audiovisual Activities

a) Blue-Hill Educational Systems, Inc.: "The Heart," Tape XIIB. This video tape lecture outlines the precordial landmarks and underlying organs. Characteristics of PMI are emphasized during discussion of inspection and palpation of precordium. The presentation includes examples of abnormal pulsations.

b) Concept Media: "Physical Assessment: Heart and Lungs," Tapes 5 and 6. Audio and filmstrip presentation describing initial assessment of cardiac function and inspection and palpation of the precordium.

c) Westinghouse Learning Health Services: "Examination of the Heart." This filmstrip and audiocassette series concentrates on the knowledge and skills of cardiac assessment. Anatomy of the heart is related to landmarks and reference lines; examination techniques are described, and characteristics of PMI are outlined.

Supplemental Activity

The following activity is suggested to strengthen your learning.

a) Frank and Alvarez-Mena: *Cardiovascular Physical Diagnosis*, "Inspection for Diseases of the Cardiovascular System," pp. 30–32, and "Palpation of the Precordium," pp. 42–47. These sections provide a direct and simple approach to signs and symptoms of cardiovascular diagnosis. Questions are included with each area to enable the reader to evaluate progress.

SELF-TEST

This Self-Test is for you. Use it to check how well you have learned the material presented in the unit. The answers follow the test.

Mark the following statements True or False.

1. _______ The anterior cardiac surface is composed primarily of the right ventricle.

2. _______ The apical pulse is produced by the right ventricle.

3. _______ Proper examination of the precordium requires that the patient be naked to the waist.

4. _______ The pulmonary arteries, aorta and atria are referred to as the base of the heart.

5. _______ The left atrium forms the right border of the anterior cardiac surface.

6. The_______________ is located parallel to and midway between the midsternal line and the acromioclavicular joint.

7. The anterior axillary line is (diagonal/perpendicular) to the anterior axillary fold.

8. Pulsations on the precordium are normally seen only at the _______________ .

9. Adults with increased cardiac output due to anxiety, anemia and fever may have a slight palpable _______________ _______________ impulse as well as an apical impulse.

10. In very thin normal individuals epigastric pulsations may be visible. These palpations are produced by the _______________ .

Identify the following areas on the accompanying drawing.

11. _______ Aortic area

12. _______ Erb's point

13. _______ Tricuspid area

14. _______ Pulmonary area

15. _______ Apical area

16. The normal apical impulse is located at
    a) the 5th intercostal space at the left sternal border.
    b) the 2nd intercostal space at the right sternal border.
    c) the 5th intercostal space 7–9 cm left of the sternal border.
    d) the right of the xiphoid process.

17. The size or diameter of the apical impulse is normally
    a) 0.05 to 0.10 cm.
    b) 0.15 to 0.25 cm.
    c) 1.0 to 2.0 cm.
    d) 3.0 to 4.0 cm.

18. The amplitude of the apical impulse is normally
    a) forceful and thrusting.
    b) light or even absent.
    c) increased with cardiac failure.
    d) unaffected by excitement.

19. In left ventricular hypertrophy the duration of the apical impulse lasts
    a) less than one-half of systole.
    b) up to two-thirds of systole.

    c) throughout systole.

    d) throughout systole and diastole.

20. A thrill is best defined as a
    a) palpable cardiac murmur.
    b) retraction of the rib cage.
    c) pulsation located above the third rib.
    d) pulsation located below the third rib.

SELF-TEST KEY

1. True. The largest portion of the anterior surface of the heart is composed of the right ventricle. The right atrium occupies a small area to the extreme right, and the left ventricle a small area to the extreme left.

2. False. The apical impulse located normally in the 5th left intercostal space slightly medial to the midclavicular line is produced by the contraction of the left ventricle.

3. True. During examination of the chest, the anterior chest is exposed and tangential lighting is used to see any pulsations emanating from the heart and great vessels. The female breasts may be covered intermittently by a towel to preserve modesty.

4. True. The base of the heart is defined as the general area occupied by the roots of the great vessels and the atria; it is directed upward and to the right.

5. False. The left atrium forms a small portion of the superior left border of the heart. Normally it cannot be examined directly because of its predominantly posterior position. The right border of the heart is formed by the right atrium.

6. Midclavicular line (MCL). By definition the MCL is a vertical line parallel to and midway between the midsternal line and the outer end of the clavicle.

7. Perpendicular. The anterior axillary line is an imaginary line drawn at a right angle from the anterior axillary fold. It is utilized as a landmark to localize and describe physical findings on the chest.

8. Apex. Normally precordial pulsations are seen only at the apex. It is also true that an apical impulse will be seen in only about half of the normal adult population.

9. Right ventricular. Increased cardiac output accentuates the amplitude and duration of cardiac impulse. Thus, slight right ventricular as well as apical impulses may be palpated in persons with fever, hyperthyroidism, anemia or anxiety.

10. Aorta. The aorta descends through the posterior mediastinum. In very thin normal individuals or persons with fever, anemia or hyperthyroidism, pulsations may be observed in the epigastric area.

11. (e) The aortic area is located in the second intercostal space to the right of the sternum.

12. (b) Erb's point is located in the secondary aortic area in the third intercostal space to the left of the sternum.

13. (c) The tricuspid area is located at the lower left sternal border.

14. (a) The pulmonary area is located in the second intercostal space to the left of the sternum.

15. (d) The apical area is normally in the fifth intercostal space just medial to the midclavicular line.

16. (c) The apical impulse or PMI (point of maximal impulse) is normally located in the fifth intercostal space 7–9 cm from the left sternal border. Normal variations such as deep inspiration, pregnancy and obesity will move the PMI to the left; very tall, thin individuals may have a PMI less than 7 cm from the sternal border.

17. (c) The size of the apical impulse is normally 1 to 2 cm or less.

18. (b) The amplitude of the normal apical impulse is felt as a light tapping. In over half the normal adult population it will not be palpable.

19. (c) In left ventricular hypertrophy the amplitude of the PMI is more forceful, it is usually displaced downward and to the left, its diameter is greater than 2 cm and it usually lasts throughout systole.

20. (a) Thrills are palpable vibrations or murmurs which are produced by turbulent blood flow through narrowed or restricted heart valves.

CLINICAL COMPONENT

The Clinical Component for Units 17 through 19 is presented in Unit 20, The Cardiovascular System: Clinical Component. Preview the Clinical Objectives in that unit and the Performance Guide cards for inspection and palpation of the precordium located in Appendix II. Facilitate your learning by practicing these skills before proceeding to the next unit.

PRE-TEST

UNIT 18

1. Which of the following statements best describes the function of the diaphragm of a stethoscope?
   a) The diaphragm is used to accentuate low-frequency sounds.
   b) The diaphragm should be used to auscultate gallop rhythms.
   c) The diaphragm is used to accentuate high-frequency sounds.
   d) For maximum efficiency, the diaphragm should be pressed very lightly against the skin.

2. Generally, cardiac auscultation is done with the client
   a) in a sitting position.
   b) in the supine position.
   c) in the left lateral position.
   d) in the upright position.

3. The first heart sound (S_1) is attributed to
   a) closure of the semilunar valves.
   b) closure of the mitral valve.
   c) opening of the semilunar valves.
   d) closure of the atrioventricular valves.

4. Which of the following is *not* a characteristic of physiological splitting?
   a) Splitting is normal in children and adolescents.
   b) Splitting is best heard at the pulmonary area and Erb's point.
   c) Splitting is best heard during expiration.
   d) Splitting is best appreciated toward the end of inspiration.

5. The two components of the second heart sound (S_2) are
   a) M_1 and T_1.
   b) M_1 and A_2.
   c) T_1 and P_2.
   d) A_2 and P_2.

6. Which of the following is *not* an auscultatory characteristic of S_1?
   a) S_1 is normally heard loudest at the apex.
   b) Anemia, exercise and hyperthyroidism tend to increase the intensity of S_1.
   c) Splitting of S_1 in normal subjects may be heard over the tricuspid area.
   d) Under normal circumstances the T_1 is louder than M_1.

7. The base of the heart is auscultated at
   a) the aortic and pulmonary areas.
   b) the aortic area and Erb's point.
   c) the pulmonary area and tricuspid area.
   d) the apical area and left sternal border.

8. The normal fourth heart sound (S_4) is a low frequency sound which is generated by
   a) rapid filling of the atria.
   b) rapid filling of the ventricles.
   c) atrial contraction.
   d) ventricular contraction.

9. An accentuated second heart sound (S_2) may be due to
   a) increased distance of heart from chest wall, as in COPD.
   b) administration of epinephrine.
   c) thyrotoxicosis.
   d) systemic or pulmonary hypertension.

10. Which of the following is important to remember when timing cardiac events?
    1. Diastole is longer than systole.
    2. Diastole is shorter than systole.
    3. S_1 has a longer duration and lower tone than S_2.
    4. S_2 is of shorter duration and higher pitch than S_1.
    5. S_2 is heard best at the apex.
    6. S_2 is louder at the aortic and pulmonary areas.
    a) 2, 3 and 6 are correct.
    b) 1, 3, 4 and 5 are correct.
    c) 1, 3, 4 and 6 are correct.
    d) 2, 4 and 6 are correct.

Indicate whether statements 11 through 15 are True (a) or False (b).

11. _______ An S_3 heard in an adult is called a ventricular gallop and is indicative of disease.

12. _______ Mitral insufficiency will increase the intensity of S_1 because of the shortened chordae tendineae and fibrosis of papillary muscles.

13. _______ A variable S_1 is heard with atrial fibrillation.

14. _______ When the loudness of P_2 equals or exceeds the loudness of A_2 pulmonary hypertension should be suspected.

15. _______ The bell of the stethoscope should be applied lightly to auscultate low-frequency sounds.

Match the following terms with the definitions in items 16 through 20.

   a) Paradoxical splitting
   b) Summation gallop
   c) Fixed splitting
   d) A_2
   e) P_2

16. _______ Under normal circumstances it is the softer component of the second heart sound (S_2).

17. _______ It is due to delayed closure of the aortic valve secondary to aortic stenosis or left bundle branch block.

18. ______ Under normal circumstances it is the louder component of S_2 that can be heard over the entire precordium.

19. ______ It does not vary with inspiration or expiration and is commonly found with atrial septal defects.

20. ______ It occurs when S_3 and S_4 are present with a heart rate of 100 or more.

Number 18

Examination of the Cardiovascular System—Auscultation

RATIONALE

The purpose of this self-instructional unit is to help you learn cardiac auscultation. The unit concentrates on evaluating heart sounds in the five auscultatory areas. At the end of this unit you will be able to differentiate between first and second heart sounds at each of the auscultatory areas, describe your findings and make judgments regarding their normality or abnormality.

GLOSSARY OF TERMS

Review the following terms before beginning this unit. You should be able to define or describe them readily.

Aortic insufficiency ____

Aortic stenosis ____

Aortic valve closure sound (A_2) ____

Atrial gallop (S_4) ____

Bell (stethoscope) ____

Bradycardia ____

Coarctation of aorta ____

Diaphragm (stethoscope) ____

First heart sound (S_1) ____

Friction rub ____

Gallop rhythm ____

Inching ____

Mitral insufficiency ____

Mitral stenosis ____

Mitral valve closure sound (M_1) _______________________________

Paradoxical splitting ____

Physiological splitting ____

Pulmonary insufficiency ____

Pulmonary stenosis ____

Pulmonic valve closure sound (P_2) ______________________________

Second heart sound (S_2) _______________________________________

Split sound ____

Summation gallop ____

Tachycardia ____

Third heart sound (S_3) ____

Tricuspid insufficiency ____

Tricuspid stenosis ____

Tricuspid valve closure sound (T_1) ______________________________

COGNITIVE OBJECTIVES

After completing this unit, you will be able to:

1. Explain the physiological basis of normal heart sounds.

2. Describe the duration and intensity of first and second heart sounds at the apex, right ventricular area, Erb's point, pulmonic area and aortic area.

3. List two conditions which increase the intensity of S_1.

4. List two causes of decreased intensity of S_1.

5. List two conditions which produce a variable S_1.

6. Identify the auscultatory area in which splitting of S_1 is normally heard.

7. Identify the condition in which a split S_1 is abnormal.

8. Explain the physiological basis for splitting of S_2 at the pulmonic area.

9. Describe the pathophysiological basis for abnormally wide splitting, fixed splitting and paradoxical splitting.

10. List two instances in which there is an increase in the intensity of S_2.

11. Describe the auscultatory characteristics of S_3.
     a. Intensity of sound.
     b. Area in which it is heard.
     c. Use of bell or diaphragm of stethoscope.

12. Differentiate the physiological basis of S_3 as a normal phenomenon and as an abnormal phenomenon.

13. Describe the auscultatory characteristics of S_4.
     a. Intensity of sound.
     b. Area of auscultation.
     c. Use of bell or diaphragm of stethoscope.

14. Describe the physiological basis for a gallop rhythm.

LEARNING ACTIVITIES

The Learning Activities contain the information necessary for meeting the Cognitive Objectives. Select one and proceed to work with it until you have mastered the material. Use the Cognitive Objectives as a study guide. A Self-Test is provided so that you can check how much you know. If you have difficulty with the Self-Test, please review the material in this unit.

Reading Activities

a) Bates: *A Guide to Physical Examination*, "The Heart." This chapter relates heart sounds to cardiac events, outlines examination procedures and discusses normal and abnormal heart sounds. It is well diagrammed and easy to read.

b) Delp and Manning: *Major's Physical Diagnosis*, "The Cardiovascular System – Auscultation of the Heart." The beginning student may have some difficulty in locating the necessary information in this chapter. The duration and intensity of the first and second heart sounds at the different auscultatory areas are not described. The authors have included quotations from early investigators which provide an interesting historical perspective on cardiac auscultation.

c) DeGowin and DeGowin: *Bedside Diagnostic Examination*, "The Heart – Heart Sounds." Heart sounds are related to cardiac events throughout the reading. Inching of the stethoscope is described but not the use of the bell and diaphragm. Additional readings on the characteristics of S_3 and S_4 are recommended.

d) Gillies and Alyn: *Patient Assessment and Management by the Nurse Practitioner*, "Auscultation," "Heart Sounds" and "Events of the Cardiac Cycle." Many of the salient facts related to auscultatory techniques and heart sounds are presented in this reading. Those familiar with cardiac auscultation will find this presentation a sufficient review. However, beginning students will need additional readings in order to meet the Cognitive Objectives.

e) Judge and Zuidema: *Methods of Clinical Examination: A Physiologic Approach*, "Auscultation." Each of the Cognitive Objectives is clearly presented in this reading. Heart sounds are diagrammed and explained physiologically.

f) Prior and Silberstein: *Physical Diagnosis*, "The Cardiovascular System – Auscultation." Techniques of auscultation, origin of heart sounds and their relation to cardiac events, and normal and abnormal heart sounds are thoroughly presented in this chapter.

g) Sana and Judge: *Physical Appraisal Methods in Nursing Practice*, "Physical Appraisal of Circulatory Function – Auscultation." This chapter clearly describes techniques of auscultation and outlines some common difficulties encountered by the beginning practitioner. The discussion of normal auscultatory findings is good; discussion of common abnormalities is very brief. Additional reading is recommended.

h) Sherman and Fields: *Guide to Patient Evaluation*, "The Heart – Auscultation." Complete information for meeting the Cognitive Objectives is not presented in this reading. The presentation is designed to provide a foundation in auscultatory techniques from which the beginning practitioner can extend knowledge and skills with future study.

Audiovisual Activities

a) Blue-Hill Educational Systems, Inc.: "The Heart – Part 12C." This 60-minute video tape lecture presents information on the physiology of the heart and origin of heart sounds. The lecture includes a discussion of normal and abnormal heart sounds which the lecturer relates to varying cardiac events or dysfunctions.

b) Concept Media: "Auscultation of Heart Sounds." This filmstrip presentation with accompanying audiocassette or records discusses the origins of heart sounds and relates them to cardiac events. The program includes auscultatory techniques and some common abnormalities; emphasis is on normal features.

c) Thiokel-Humetrics Corporation: "Heart Sounds: What They Teach Us" by Antonio C. deLeon, Jr. In this audiotape presentation with accompanying manual use of the stethoscope, anatomy and physiology of the heart, origin of heart sounds and examples of normal and abnormal heart sounds are presented.

d) Westinghouse Learning Health Services: "Examination of the Heart." This audio-cassette-filmstrip presentation describes the characteristics of normal heart sounds, identifies auscultatory areas and describes common abnormalities.

Supplemental Activities

The following activities are suggested to broaden or strengthen your learning.

a) Frank and Alvarez-Mena: *Cardiovascular Physical Diagnosis*. The authors discuss normal and abnormal heart sounds in a modified programmed instruction format.

b) American Heart Association: *Examination of the Heart*, "Auscultation." A pamphlet which diagrams and describes normal and abnormal heart sounds.

SELF-TEST

This Self-Test is for you. Use it to check how well you have learned the material presented in the unit. The answers follow the test.

1. The first heart sound (S_1) is produced by
    a) closure of the AV valves at the start of ventricular systole.
    b) closure of the AV valves at the beginning of diastole.
    c) opening of the semilunar valves.
    d) opening of the AV valves at the start of ventricular systole.

2. Which of the following sounds is produced by closure of the semilunar valves?
    a) first heart sound (S_1)
    b) second heart sound (S_2)

    c)   third heart sound (S_3)
    d)   fourth heart sound (S_4)

3. Ventricular systole occurs
    a)   when blood is pumped out of the ventricles.
    b)   between the first and second heart sounds.
    c)   following the second heart sound.
    d)   during both a and c.
    e)   during both a and b.

Identify the features listed in 4 through 14 as being characteristics of the first heart sound (A) or second heart sound (B).

4. ______ longer duration and lower tonal quality (lubb)

5. ______ greater intensity at the apex

6. ______ shorter duration and higher pitch (dupp)

7. ______ produced by closure of semilunar valves

8. ______ marks the beginning of diastole

9. ______ louder in the aortic and pulmonary areas

10. ______ exercise, anemia or thyrotoxicosis may increase intensity of this sound

11. ______ composed of A_2 and P_2

12. ______ systemic hypertension will increase intensity

13. ______ decreased intensity in COPD, obesity and heart failure

14. ______ AV dissociation will cause it to become variable in intensity

15. Physiological splitting is best appreciated toward the end of (inspiration/expiration).

16. Which of the following is *not* a characteristic of paradoxical splitting?
    a)   It occurs during inspiration.
    b)   It occurs during expiration.
    c)   It occurs with prolonged contraction of the left ventricle secondary to LBBB (left bundle branch block).
    d)   It occurs with delayed aortic valve closure due to aortic stenosis.

17. The third heart sound (S_3) occurs with rapid ventricular filling. It is commonly auscultated in _____________ but may indicate myocardial disease in _____________ persons.

18. The S_4 is a very soft, low-pitched sound which is best heard with the_____________ of the stethoscope.

19. In a gallop rhythm the S_1 is preceded by an _______________ and the S_2 is followed by an _______________.

20. The development of an S_3 in a patient with diagnosed myocardial infarction would indicate _______________.

SELF-TEST KEY

1. (a) The first heart sound or S_1 is produced by the closure of the AV valves at the beginning of ventricular systole. Rapid filling of the ventricle and isometric contraction of the ventricular muscle result in a rapid rise of pressure in the ventricles which exceeds atrial pressures, forcing the closure of the tricuspid and mitral valves.

2. (b) Closure of the semilunar (aortic and pulmonic) valves produces the second heart sound, or S_2. It marks the beginning of ventricular diastole.

3. (e) Ventricular contraction or systole corresponds with ventricular ejection which occurs between the first and second heart sounds.

4. (a) First heart sound. The vibrations produced by the closure of the AV valves have a lower frequency range than the vibrations resulting from closure of the semilunar valves. This results in the perception of a lower tonal quality. The longer duration is due to the asynchronous closing of the tricuspid and mitral valves.

5. (a) The closure of the AV valves causes blood to rebound in the ventricles. The vibrations transmitted to the chest wall by these phenomena are best percussed at the apex, which is the point in the precordium nearest the origin of the vibrations.

6. (b) The semilunar valves, particularly the aortic valve, close with greater force than the AV valves; this increases the frequency of vibrations and results in a higher tone, or pitch. The aortic component is the loudest component of S_2 and is transmitted widely over the precordium. Consequently, as a rule, it is the aortic component that is heard and accounts for a shorter second sound.

7. (b) The closure of the semilunar valves produces the high-pitched second heart sound.

8. (b) Diastole begins with the second heart sound, which marks the closure of the semilunar valves and initiation of ventricular relaxation.

9. (b) Sound is transmitted to the precordium at a point nearest its origin. The semilunar valves are located at the base of the heart, and the vibrations accompanying their closure are transmitted along the great vessels.

10. (a) Hyperkinetic conditions such as hyperthyroidism may increase or accentuate the S_1. These conditions tend to increase the tone of the ventricular muscle.

11. (b) The second heart sound results from the closure of the aortic (A_2) and pulmonary (P_2) semilunar valves.

12. (b) Systemic hypertension increases the back pressure exerted on the aortic leaflets. The phenomenon increases the violence with which the leaflets are closed and results in an accentuation of the sound produced.

13. (a) The first heart sound is diminished when the distance between the origin of the sound (AV valves) and the chest wall is increased (e.g., in obesity, hyperinflated lungs). Likewise, a weakened myocardium will produce sounds of lower frequency than a healthy myocardium.

14. (a) The intensity of the first heart sound is dependent upon (1) the amount of blood available for ventricular ejection and (2) the position of the AV valves at the start of ventricular systole. In AV dissociation, atrial and ventricular contractions are not synchronous. Consequently, when atrial contraction proceeds ventricular contraction by a shorter than normal P-R interval the first sound is accentuated; but when the P-R interval is extended the first sound is diminished.

15. Inspiration. Physiological splitting of the P_2 is attributed to increased venous return to the right ventricle during inspiration. The process prolongs right ventricular systole and pulmonary valve closure.

16. (a) Physiological splitting is associated with inspiration. Paradoxical splitting is characterized by splitting of the second sound during expiration and a single sound during inspiration. It is always abnormal and is due either to delayed left ventricular conduction as in left bundle-branch block or to prolonged emptying of the left ventricle as in aortic stenosis.

17. children; middle-aged. The S_3 is a faint, low-pitched sound best heard with the bell of the stethoscope, at the apex, with the client in a left lateral position. It is an extremely common finding in children and young adults but seldom heard in persons over 30. The presence of this finding in middle-aged or older individuals should alert the practitioner to the possibility of ventricular overloading or decreased myocardial contractility.

18. bell. Low-pitched sounds are best auscultated using the bell of the stethoscope. The bell tends to amplify these sounds, while the diaphragm tends to mask low-frequency sounds.

19. S_4; S_3. A gallop rhythm refers to that auscultatory phenomenon in which three and occasionally four heart sounds are present; the sound perceived by the listener resembles a horse's gallop. The S_4 that precedes S_1 is called a presystolic sound. It results from the forceful contraction of enlarged atria. The S_3 is a protodiastolic, or early diastolic, sound following S_2 and is the result of rapid ventricular filling.

20. myocardial failure. The occurrence of the third heart sound of S_3 in association with a diagnosed myocardial infarction implies ensuing cardiac failure.

CLINICAL COMPONENT

The Clinical Component for Units 17 through 19 is presented in Unit 20, The Cardiovascular System: Clinical Component. Preview the Clinical Objectives in that unit and the Performance Guide cards in Appendix II for auscultation of the precordium. Facilitate your learning by practicing these skills before proceeding to the next unit.

PRE-TEST

UNIT 19

1. The opening snap
   a) is commonly caused by mitral stenosis.
   b) is a diastolic extracardiac sound.
   c) is a systolic extracardiac sound.
   d) is described in both a and b.
   e) is described in both a and c.

2. A pericardial friction rub
   1. may occur with pericarditis and myocardial infarction.
   2. is a low-pitched humming sound heard throughout systole and diastole.
   3. is a high-pitched grating sound associated with atrial systole, ventricular systole and ventricular diastole.
   4. is best heard with the diaphragm of the stethoscope.
   5. is heard only at the apex.
   a) 1, 2 and 4 are correct.
   b) 2, 4 and 5 are correct.
   c) 1, 3 and 4 are correct.
   d) 2 and 5 are correct.

3. Cardiac murmurs
   a) are short auditory vibrations due to increased velocity of blood flow.
   b) are produced by structural or hemodynamic changes or both in the heart or great vessels.
   c) do not vary in timing or pitch.
   d) are heard best with the diaphragm of the stethoscope.

4. A diastolic murmur
   a) begins with the onset of S_1 and terminates after S_2.
   b) begins with S_2 and terminates with or before S_1.
   c) begins with the onset of S_1 and terminates before S_2.
   d) is frequently a functional or "innocent" murmur.

5. The intensity or loudness of a murmur is graded on a scale of I through VI. A loud murmur associated with a thrill would be graded as
   a) II.
   b) III.
   c) IV.
   d) V.

6. Transmission or radiation of a murmur is dependent upon
   a) the intensity of the murmur at its primary site.
   b) direction of blood flow.
   c) the distance between the source of the murmur and the chest wall.
   d) both a and c.
   e) all of the above.

7. The ejection sound or ejection click
   a) occurs early in systole.
   b) is a high-pitched sound of short duration.
   c) is a low-pitched sound of variable duration.
   d) is described in both a and b.
   e) is described in both a and c.

8. Mr. Sand is a 23-yr-old male with mitral insufficiency due to rheumatic fever. Mr. Sand has developed a holosystolic or pansystolic murmur. The holosystolic murmur of mitral insufficiency
   a) has a high-pitched, blowing quality which begins with S_1 and terminates with S_2.
   b) has a high-pitched blowing quality which begins with S_2 and terminates before S_1.
   c) has a crescendo-decrescendo quality.
   d) is preceded by an opening snap.

9. You would expect the murmur of mitral insufficiency to radiate
   a) to the neck.
   b) to the left axilla.
   c) only over the precordium.
   d) very little.

10. The pathophysiological mechanism underlying the murmur in mitral insufficiency is
    a) blood flow across a partial obstruction.
    b) left-to-right shunting.
    c) abrupt dilatation of the aorta.
    d) backflow of blood from the left ventricle into the left atrium.

11. Aortic stenosis produces a
    a) diastolic decrescendo murmur.
    b) midsystolic ejection murmur.
    c) holosystolic murmur.
    d) crescendo-decrescendo diastolic murmur.

12. Kathy D. has been admitted to the cardiac unit for repair of a ventricular septal defect. You would describe her heart murmur as
    1. holosystolic.
    2. holodiastolic.
    3. loudest at the left sternal border.
    4. radiating into the left axilla.
    5. high pitched and heard best with the diaphragm.
    a) 1, 3 and 4 are correct.
    b) 2, 4 and 5 are correct.
    c) 1, 3 and 5 are correct.
    d) 2, 3, 4 and 5 are correct.

13. Shunting of blood from a high-pressure chamber such as an artery into a low-pressure chamber such as a vein produces
    a) a continuous murmur which has a humming quality.
    b) a continuous murmur which has a crescendo-decrescendo quality.
    c) a grating sound corresponding to cardiac contraction.
    d) an ejection click.

14. Mrs. Jones has stated that she has a heart murmur. On auscultation you discover a rumbling diastolic murmur preceded by an opening snap. Mrs. Jones probably has
    a) aortic stenosis.
    b) mitral stenosis.
    c) aortic insufficiency.
    d) mitral insufficiency.

15. Mrs. Jones' murmur is heard best
    a) with the bell of the stethoscope.
    b) with the diaphragm of the stethoscope.
    c) with Mrs. Jones in the left lateral position.
    d) when both a and c are used.
    e) when both b and c are used.

16. The blowing diastolic murmur of aortic regurgitation is due to
    a) dilatation of the mitral rings.
    b) regurgitation of blood from the left ventricle into the left atrium.
    c) blood flow across a deformed or dilated aortic valve.
    d) left-to-right shunting.

17. The diastolic murmur of aortic regurgitation
    a) tends to be loudest with the client sitting and leaning forward.
    b) begins after S_2 and then diminishes.
    c) has a very high pitch.
    d) is described by all of the above.

18. Mrs. Firth has come to the clinic for a prenatal check up. On auscultating her heart you note a grade II midsystolic ejection murmur which was not there before. Mrs. Firth has complaints of fatigue and occasional palpitations. Her hemoglobin is 8.5 gm. Mrs. Firth's murmur is probably
    a) an early sign of aortic stenosis.
    b) an "innocent" or functional murmur.
    c) due to mitral insufficiency.
    d) due to a congenital anomaly.

19. Mrs. Firth's heart murmur may be related to
    a) an increase in stroke volume due to anemia.
    b) blood flow through an incompetent valve.
    c) blood flow across a stenosed tricuspid valve.
    d) rapid ventricular filling.

20. Mr. Rush has had a myocardial infarction. On the second day of hospitalization he develops a pericardial friction rub. The high-pitched grating noises associated with pericardial friction rubs
    a) vary with respirations.
    b) are composed of a systolic component only.
    c) are frequently confused with murmurs.
    d) are produced by the back-and-forth movement of the pericardial surfaces over each other.

Number 19

Abnormal Cardiac Sounds: Murmurs and Friction Rubs

RATIONALE

This self-instructional unit is designed to introduce you to auscultation of abnormal heart sounds, cardiac murmurs and pericardial friction rubs. This unit focuses on understanding the pathophysiological mechanisms behind the production of these abnormal cardiac transmissions. At the end of this unit you will demonstrate knowledge of abnormal heart sounds, cardiac murmurs and pericardial friction rubs by your ability to systematically describe each abnormal heart sound according to its occurrence in the cardiac cycle, location on precordium, intensity, pitch, radiation of transmission and quality.

GLOSSARY OF TERMS

Review the following terms before and after completing this unit. You should be able to define or describe them readily.

Aortic regurgitation ____

Ejection click ____

Functional or innocent murmur ______________________________________

Holodiastolic ____

Holosystolic ____

Midsystolic ____

Middiastolic ____

Opening snap ____

Patent ductus arteriosus ____

Pericardial friction rub ____

Presystolic ____

Protodiastolic ____

Ventricular septal defect ____

COGNITIVE OBJECTIVES

At the end of this unit you will demonstrate knowledge of abnormal heart sounds, cardiac murmurs and pericardial friction rubs by your ability to:

1. Differentiate between ejection clicks and opening snaps according to their
   a. origin of sound.
   b. timing in cardiac cycle.
   c. location on precordium.
   d. pitch – low, medium, high.

2. Describe at least four pathophysiological mechanisms which favor the production of murmurs within the heart or great vessels.

3. Recall and define the six categories which describe cardiac murmurs.
   a. Timing – systolic, diastolic, continuous.
   b. Location – described in terms of anatomical landmarks or interspace.
   c. Intensity – grade I to grade VI.
   d. Pitch – low, medium, high.
   e. Radiation – transmission of sound on precordium.
   f. Quality – crescendo, decrescendo, harsh, rumbling, musical, blowing.

4. Explain what is meant by the term functional or "innocent" murmur.

5. Distinguish between midsystolic ejection murmurs and holosystolic regurgitant murmurs according to their
   a. direction of blood flow.
   b. time.
   c. location.
   d. intensity.
   e. pitch.
   f. radiation.
   g. quality.
   h. common pathophysiological causes.

6. Discuss the differences between diastolic murmurs caused by semilunar valve insufficiency and those caused by atrioventricular valve stenosis in regard to
   a. time.
   b. location.
   c. intensity.
   d. pitch.
   e. radiation.
   f. quality.

7. Delineate the characteristics and pathophysiological causes of continuous murmurs.

8. Outline and describe the auscultatory components of pericardial friction rubs.

LEARNING ACTIVITIES

The Learning Activities each contain the information necessary for meeting the Cognitive Objectives. Select one and proceed to work with it until you have mastered the material. Use the Cognitive Objectives as a study guide. A Self-Test is provided so that you can check how much you know. If you have difficulty with the Self-Test, please review the material in this unit.

Reading Activities

a) Bates: *A Guide to Physical Examination*, "The Heart." In this chapter the author has accompanied each description of abnormal heart sounds with an illustration showing blood flow. This reading offers a concise, clear presentation of information.

b) Delp and Manning: *Major's Physical Diagnosis*, "The Cardiovascular System," pp. 430–458. This chapter provides a thorough description of pathophysiological mechanism underlying production of abnormal heart sounds and murmurs. Characteristics of murmurs are differentiated clearly, and numerous illustrations facilitate understanding.

c) DeGowin and DeGowin: *Bedside Diagnostic Examination*, "Auscultation of Cardiac Murmurs." This advanced and greatly detailed discussion of cardiac murmurs associated with various cardiac dysfunctions is not suggested for the beginning student.

d) Gillies and Alyn: *Physical Assessment and Management by the Nurse Practitioner*, "The Physical Examination," pp. 84–86. An overview of the pathophysiological mechanisms which result in the production of vibrations associated with cardiac murmurs is presented. Discussion is quite brief, and additional readings are suggested.

e) Judge and Zuidema: *Methods of Clinical Examination: A Physiologic Approach*, "Circulatory System," pp. 181–191. Abnormal heart sounds are clearly described and illustrated. Presentation is concise and readable.

f) Prior and Silberstein: *Physical Diagnosis*, "The Cardiovascular System," pp. 268–281. Abnormal heart sounds are discussed and related to underlying cardiac pathophysiology. Auscultatory techniques are reviewed and applied to identifying characteristics of cardiac murmurs. Phonocardiograms are utilized to demonstrate heart sounds.

g) Sana and Judge: *Physical Appraisal Methods in Nursing Practice*, "Physical Appraisal of Circulatory Function," pp. 201–205. This chapter presents an overview of abnormal heart sounds and mechanisms which are relevant to their production. Additional readings are recommended.

h) Sherman and Fields: *Guide to Patient Evaluation*, "The Heart." Categories of heart murmurs are well described. A table of common heart murmurs outlines characteristics of systolic and diastolic murmurs. The information is presented simply, providing a good introduction for the neophyte.

Audiovisual Activities

a) Blue-Hill Educational Systems, Inc.: "Cardiovascular System – Part XIID." This 30-minute videocassette lecture presents material on the pathophysiological origin of cardiac murmurs, describes their characteristics, discusses systolic and diastolic murmurs and differentiates between functional and dysfunctional murmurs.

b) Concept Media: *Physical Assessment: Heart and Lungs*, "Auscultation of Heart Sounds." Filmstrips and audiocassettes are utilized to describe normal and common abnormal heart sounds.

c) Thiokol-Humetrics: *Heart Sounds: What They Teach Us*. This audiocassette series with accompanying book describes and presents examples of abnormal heart sounds. It provides an in-depth presentation.

d) Westinghouse Learning Health Service: "Examination of the Heart." This filmstrip audiocassette module includes authentic heart sounds. Emphasis is on recognition and description of abnormal heart sounds.

Supplemental Activities

a) American Heart Association: "Auscultation." This pamphlet provides illustrations and descriptions of normal and abnormal heart sounds.

b) Merck, Sharp and Dohme: "Cardiac Auscultation." Audiocassettes and records present normal and abnormal heart sounds produced by cardiac simulator.

c) Frank and Alvarez-Mena: *Cardiovascular Physical Diagnosis*. This modified program instruction is designed to assist the student in developing skills in cardiac auscultation.

SELF-TEST

This Self-Test is for you. Use it to check how well you have learned the material presented in this unit. The answers follow the test.

1. Ejection clicks
    a) occur during systole.
    b) occur during diastole.
    c) are generated by abrupt distention of aorta or pulmonary artery.
    d) are described in both a and c.
    e) are described in both b and c.

2. Opening snaps can be differentiated from ejection clicks by
    a) their timing in the cardiac cycle.
    b) their location (heard only at left sternal border).
    c) the fact that they vary with respiration.
    d) the fact that they do not radiate.

3. The pathophysiological mechanisms underlying the production of heart murmurs include
    1. increased velocity of blood flow.
    2. decreased velocity of blood flow.
    3. blood flow across a partial obstruction.
    4. blood flow into a dilated chamber.
    5. regurgitant flow across an incompetent valve or other defect.
    a) 2, 3, 4 and 5 are correct.
    b) 1, 3, 4 and 5 are correct.
    c) 3 and 5 are correct.
    d) 3, 4 and 5 are correct.

4. Systolic murmurs
    a) begin with or after S_2 and end before or at S_1.
    b) begin in systole and continue into or throughout diastole.
    c) begin with or after S_1 and end at or before S_2.
    d) are confined to the period just prior to the initiation of S_1.

5. A grade II/VI murmur is
    a) so faint that it can hardly be heard.

   b) faint but can be recognized readily.
   c) moderately loud.
   d) loud and associated with a thrill.

6. The location of a murmur is
   a) the area to which it radiates.
   b) the area of the precordium at which it is loudest.
   c) determined by inching of the stethoscope.
   d) of little diagnostic value.

7. Holosystolic murmurs are
   1. due to backflow of blood from ventricles to atria across incompetent AV valves.
   2. due to obstructed blood flow through stenotic AV valves.
   3. heard throughout systole.
   4. auscultated when there is a left-to-right shunt through a ventricular septal defect.
   5. heard after S_2.
   a) 1, 2 and 3 are correct.
   b) 2, 4 and 5 are correct.
   c) 1, 3 and 4 are correct.
   d) 4 and 5 are correct.

8. Diastolic murmurs
   a) are always indicative of heart disease.
   b) are usually functional or "innocent" murmurs.
   c) result from AV valve stenosis or semilunar valve incompetence.
   d) are described in both b and c.
   e) are described in both a and c.

9. Pericardial friction rubs
   a) radiate over the entire precordium.
   b) are triphasic grating noises auscultated in the presence of pericarditis.
   c) have a humming or roaring quality.
   d) are very low pitched.

10. Continuous murmurs
   a) occur in both systole and diastole.
   b) have a crescendo-decrescendo quality.
   c) result from an abnormal communication between the arterial and venous circulations.
   d) are described in all of the above.

Match the following conditions with the abnormal cardiac sounds or murmurs they produce.

11. _______ Grade I and II murmurs	a) Mitral stenosis
	b) Aortic regurgitation
12. _______ Midsystolic ejection murmur	c) Functional or "innocent" murmur
	d) Aortic stenosis
13. _______ Decrescendo diastolic murmurs	e) Pericarditis
	f) Patent ductus arteriosus
14. _______ Opening snap	

15. _______ Continuous murmur

16. _______ High-pitched grating noise

SELF-TEST KEY

1. (d) Ejection clicks occur after S_1 and before S_2 and are therefore systolic in nature; ejection clicks are generated by the abrupt dilatation of either the aortic or pulmonary artery by a sudden jet of blood against the arterial wall. The sound tends to occur with ventricular overloading due to valvular obstruction or hypertension.

2. (a) The opening snap is a diastolic sound produced by the opening of stenosed AV valves. The mitral valve is affected most commonly; the sound radiates widely and is best heard at the apex. The opening snap occurs earlier, is sharper and is higher in pitch than the S_3.

3. (b) Murmurs are produced by structural or hemodynamic changes or both in the heart or great vessels. These changes include increased velocity of blood flow, flow across partial obstructions, backflow of blood across an incompetent valve, blood flow from a high-pressure area through an abnormal passage and increased flow into a dilated chamber.

4. (c) Systole occurs between S_1 and S_2; therefore, systolic murmurs will be heard with or after S_1 and will end before S_2.

5. (b) A grade II/VI murmur is faint but readily audible. An innocent or functional systolic murmur is usually no louder than grade II.

6. (b) A loud murmur may be heard over the entire precordium but is located in the area where it is loudest, usually in one of the five auscultatory areas on the precordium.

7. (c) Holosystolic or pansystolic murmurs occur throughout systole (S_1–S_2) and are due to regurgitation of blood from the ventricles into the atria across an incompetent AV valve or through an abnormal connection between the right and left ventricles.

8. (e) Diastolic murmurs, unlike systolic murmurs, are always indicative of heart disease. Diastolic murmurs result from stenosis of an AV valve, causing a rumbling murmur during rapid ventricular filling, or from incompetence of one of the semilunar valves, producing a decrescendo murmur that begins with S_2 and ends before S_1.

9. (b) Pericardial friction rubs result from inflammation of the pericardial sac. The rub has a high-pitched, grating quality like that produced by sandpaper. The rub has three components associated with cardiac contraction: (1) atrial systole, (2) ventricular systole and (3) ventricular diastole. Friction rubs may be transient or may remain for several days.

10. (d) Continuous murmurs begin in systole and continue into diastole without stopping. They are found in conditions in which there is blood flow from a high-pressure chamber (artery) to a low-pressure chamber (vein), such as patent ductus arteriosus.

11.   (c)   Grade I and II murmurs are usually functional or "innocent" murmurs.

12.   (d)   Aortic stenosis is characterized by a midsystolic ejection murmur, which results from sudden dilatation of the aorta as blood jets through a stiff aortic valve.

13.   (b)   Aortic regurgitation is characterized by a diastolic murmur which is high-pitched and begins immediately with closure of the aortic valve and diminishes as diastole progresses (decrescendo).

14.   (a)   The opening snap occurring with mitral stenosis is a sharp click heard in diastole and is associated with opening of the stenotic valve. The higher the left atrial pressures, the closer the opening snap is to the second heart sound (S_2).

15.   (f)   Patent ductus arteriosus produces a murmur which begins in systole and continues into diastole. It has a crescendo-decrescendo quality which is usually loud, obscures S_2 and may be associated with a thrill.

16.   (e)   Pericarditis, or inflammation of the pericardial sac, produces a high-pitched, scratchy sound as the pericardium moves back and forth with cardiac contraction.

CLINICAL COMPONENT

The Clinical Component for Units 17 through 19 is presented in Unit 20, The Cardiovascular System: Clinical Component. Preview the Clinical Objectives in that unit and the Performance Guide cards in Appendix II for auscultation of the precordium. Facilitate your learning by practicing these skills before proceeding to the next unit.

Number 20

The Cardiovascular System: Clinical Component

Having completed the cognitive portion of the units on cardiovascular assessment, you are now ready to proceed to the Clinical Objectives. The purpose of the Clinical Component is to provide you with specific guidelines for the assessment of cardiac function.

CLINICAL OBJECTIVES

At the end of this unit you will perform inspection, palpation and auscultation of the precordium, correlating physical examination skills with physiological principles. You will be able to:

1. Demonstrate knowledge of normal cardiac function and of signs and symptoms of cardiac dysfunction by obtaining a pertinent health history from the client.

2. Demonstrate inspection and palpation of the precordium by assessing
   a. configuration of thorax — pectus excavatum, barrel chest, pectus carinatum, bulges on chest wall.
   b. respirations — dyspnea, tachypnea.
   c. nutritional status — adequate, obesity, cachexia.
   d. skin — color, tone, vascularity.
   e. chest wall pulsations — location, duration, amplitude, size.
      1) apical area
      2) tricuspid area
      3) Erb's point
      4) pulmonary area
      5) aortic area

3. Demonstrate cardiac auscultation by
   a. correctly positioning patient for optimal accentuation of heart sounds:
      1) supine — for all sounds
      2) left lateral — apical sounds
      3) sitting — aortic and pulmonary sounds
   b. utilizing the diaphragm and bell of the stethoscope.
   c. demonstrating "inching" of stethoscope across the auscultatory areas of the precordium.
   d. describing the intensity and duration of S_1 at the five areas of auscultation.
   e. describing the intensity and duration of S_2 at the five auscultatory areas.
   f. identifying physiological splitting of S_2 at Erb's point and/or pulmonary area.
   g. identifying S_3 and S_4 when present.

    h. identifying opening snaps and ejection clicks when present.
    i.   identifying and describing characteristics of murmurs when present.

4. Utilize S.O.A.P. to systematically describe findings, assess normality and formulate a plan of action.

INSTRUCTIONS

Utilizing three of your peers or clients in the clinical area, practice inspection, palpation and auscultation of the precordium. Remove the Performance Guide cards for Unit 20 from Appendix II. These cards will enable you to practice the skills necessary to meet the Clinical Objectives and complete the Response Sheets. On each Response Sheet you will be expected to (1) ask questions which elicit possible symptoms, (2) systematically describe your findings, (3) localize any abnormalities present and (4) summarize your examination findings using the S.O.A.P. method of recording.

EQUIPMENT

Ruler
Stethoscope with bell and diaphragm

OPTIONAL ACTIVITIES

These activities demonstrate techniques for assessment of the cardiovascular system.
a) Bates: "The Heart." This film demonstrates precordial examination techniques.
b) Blue-Hill Educational Systems, Inc.: "Cardiovascular Examination." This video tape cassette includes demonstration of peripheral and precordial examination techniques.

Client ______________________________

Date ___________________ Age _______ Sex ______

Examiner ______________________________

I. Health History

II. Physical Examination

A. Inspection

1. Configuration of the thorax

2. Respirations

3. Nutritional status

4. Skin

5. Chest wall pulsations

6. PMI (location, amplitude, size)

B. Palpation

1. Apical area (PMI)

    a. Location

    b. Amplitude

    c. Duration

    d. Size

    e. Rate

    f. Rhythm

    g. Thrills

2. Tricuspid area (pulsations, thrills, lift, heave)

3. Erb's point (pulsations, thrills)

4. Pulmonary area (pulsations, thrills)

5. Aortic area (pulsations, thrills)

C. Auscultation

Diagram heart sounds as shown here: S_1 S_2 S_3
(Height of lines indicates loudness; width indicates length of time.)

1. Apical area

    a. Intensity and duration of heart sounds

b. Abnormal heart sounds

2. Tricuspid area (intensity, duration and splitting of heart sounds)

3. Erb's point (intensity, splitting, abnormal sounds)

4. Pulmonary area (intensity, splitting, abnormal heart sounds)

5. Aortic area (intensity, splitting, abnormal heart sounds)

Summarize your findings using the S.O.A.P. method.

S. **(Client's observations, complaints, health history)**

O. **(Physical findings)**

A. **(Assessment of the problem, diagnosis)**

P. **(Plans for teaching, further evaluation, care)**

Client _______________________________________

Date _________________ Age _______ Sex _______

Examiner _____________________________________

I. Health History

II. Physical Examination

   A. Inspection

     1. Configuration of the thorax

     2. Respirations

     3. Nutritional status

     4. Skin

     5. Chest wall pulsations

     6. PMI (location, amplitude, size)

   B. Palpation

     1. Apical area (PMI)

    a. Location

    b. Amplitude

    c. Duration

    d. Size

    e. Rate

    f. Rhythm

    g. Thrills

2. Tricuspid area (pulsations, thrills, lift, heave)

3. Erb's point (pulsations, thrills)

4. Pulmonary area (pulsations, thrills)

5. Aortic area (pulsations, thrills)

C. Auscultation

Diagram heart sounds as shown here: S_1 S_2 S_3
(Height of lines indicates loudness; width indicates length of time.)

1. Apical area

    a. Intensity and duration of heart sounds

b. Abnormal heart sounds

2. Tricuspid area (intensity, duration and splitting of heart sounds)

3. Erb's point (intensity, splitting, abnormal sounds)

4. Pulmonary area (intensity, splitting, abnormal heart sounds)

5. Aortic area (intensity, splitting, abnormal heart sounds)

Summarize your findings using the S.O.A.P. method.

S. (Client's observations, complaints, health history)

O. (Physical findings)

A. (Assessment of the problem, diagnosis)

P. (Plans for teaching, further evaluation, care)

Client _______________________________________

Date ____________________ Age _______ Sex _______

Examiner _____________________________________

I. Health History

II. Physical Examination

A. Inspection

1. Configuration of the thorax

2. Respirations

3. Nutritional status

4. Skin

5. Chest wall pulsations

6. PMI (location, amplitude, size)

B. Palpation

1. Apical area (PMI)

    a. Location

    b. Amplitude

    c. Duration

    d. Size

    e. Rate

    f. Rhythm

    g. Thrills

2. Tricuspid area (pulsations, thrills, lift, heave)

3. Erb's point (pulsations, thrills)

4. Pulmonary area (pulsations, thrills)

5. Aortic area (pulsations, thrills)

C. Auscultation

Diagram heart sounds as shown here: S_1 S_2 S_3
(Height of lines indicates loudness; width indicates length of time.)

1. Apical area

    a. Intensity and duration of heart sounds

   b. Abnormal heart sounds

2. Tricuspid area (intensity, duration and splitting of heart sounds)

3. Erb's point (intensity, splitting, abnormal sounds)

4. Pulmonary area (intensity, splitting, abnormal heart sounds)

5. Aortic area (intensity, splitting, abnormal heart sounds)

Summarize your findings using the S.O.A.P. method.

S. (Client's observations, complaints, health history)

O. (Physical findings)

A. (Assessment of the problem, diagnosis)

P. (Plans for teaching, further evaluation, care)

SECTION IV

LOWER TORSO

UNIT 21

1. Parietal pain is
    1. sharp and well localized.
    2. dull and diffuse.
    3. often referred pain.
    4. due to stretching.
    5. a sign of peritoneal involvement.
    a) 2 and 4 are correct.
    b) 1, 3 and 5 are correct.
    c) 2, 3 and 4 are correct.
    d) 2 and 5 are correct.

2. The term scaphoid is used to describe an abdomen that is
    a) bulging.
    b) asymmetrical.
    c) concave.
    d) infected with scabies.

3. During assessment of the abdomen the examiner should note
    1. symmetry.
    2. rashes or lesions.
    3. prominent venous patterns.
    4. umbilical characteristics.
    5. striae.
    a) 1, 2 and 4 are correct.
    b) 1, 3 and 5 are correct.
    c) 3, 4 and 5 are correct.
    d) 3 and 5 are correct.
    e) all of the above are correct.

Match each of the structures in 4 through 8 with the quadrant in which it is located.

4. _______ Left ovary

5. _______ Gallbladder

6. _______ Spleen

7. _______ Stomach

8. _______ Appendix

a) Left upper quadrant
b) Right upper quadrant
c) Left lower quadrant
d) Right lower quadrant

9. Abnormal umbilical signs include
    1. marked eversion.
    2. discoloration.

    3. displacement.
    4. excoriation.
    5. inguinal hernia.
   a) 1, 2 and 3 are correct.
   b) 4 and 5 are correct.
   c) 1, 3 and 5 are correct.
   d) 1, 2, 3 and 4 are correct.
   e) all of the above are correct.

10. High midline abdominal pulsations of low amplitude and directed forward are probably
   a) normal aortic pulsations.
   b) borborygmi.
   c) aortic pulsations masked by an overlying mass.
   d) caused by an aortic aneurysm.
   e) caused by a partial bowel obstruction.

11. Percussion notes normally heard in the abdomen are
   a) resonance, hyperresonance, flatness.
   b) tympany, hyperresonance, dullness.
   c) resonance, dullness, tympany.
   d) flatness, resonance, dullness.
   e) resonance, hyperresonance, dullness.

12. Auscultation of the abdomen is performed after inspection because
   a) percussion and palpation distort bowel sounds.
   b) auscultation usually follows inspection.
   c) palpation may alter placement of the organs and blood vessels.
   d) percussion may be painful.

13. Deep palpation is used to assess
    1. organ size.
    2. masses.
    3. rebound tenderness.
    4. guarding.
    5. density of underlying organs and spaces.
   a) 1, 2, 3 and 5 are correct.
   b) 2, 4 and 5 are correct.
   c) 1, 2, and 5 are correct.
   d) 3 and 4 are correct.
   e) all of the above are correct.

14. Tenderness along the anterior costal margins may be a sign of
   a) kidney infection.
   b) liver or spleen enlargement.
   c) cystitis.
   d) renal calculi.
   e) appendicitis.

15. Percussion over the symphysis pubis reveals a well-delineated area of dullness. You suspect
    1. fecal material in transverse colon.
    2. pregnancy.

      3. distended bladder.
      4. hepatomegaly.
      5. normal percussion note.
   a) 1, 2 and 4 are correct.
   b) 5 only is correct.
   c) 2 and 3 are correct.
   d) 1 and 3 are correct.
   e) 4 only is correct.

16. Generalized distention of the abdomen may be noted with
      1. obesity.
      2. ectopic pregnancy.
      3. splenomegaly.
      4. ascites.
      5. cancer of the bladder.
   a) 1, 3 and 5 are correct.
   b) 2 and 3 are correct.
   c) 1 and 4 are correct.
   d) 4 only is correct.
   e) all of the above are correct.

Match each condition in 17 through 19 with its characteristic bowel sound.

17. _______ Complete bowel obstruction

18. _______ Partial obstruction

19. _______ Gastritis

   a) Absent bowel sounds
   b) Increased bowel sounds
   c) Sluggish bowel sounds

20. Liver size is measured by
   a) percussion from resonance to dullness.
   b) light palpation over the right upper quadrant.
   c) percussion along the right axillary line.
   d) deep palpation in the right lower quadrant.

Number 21

Examination of the Abdomen

RATIONALE

This self-instructional unit is designed to help you learn systematic inspection, auscultation, percussion and palpation of the abdomen. The primary emphasis is on identifying and describing the abdominal structures in relation to anatomical landmarks and recognizing common abnormalities.

GLOSSARY OF TERMS

Review these terms before and after completing this unit. You should be able to define or describe them readily.

Aneurysm __________

Ascites __________

Borborygmi __________

Bruits __________

Cecum __________

Cholecystitis __________

Costal margin __________

Costovertebral angle (CVA) __________

Diverticulitis __________

Epigastrium __________

Hepatomegaly __________

Hernia __________

Inguinal ligament __________

Linea alba __________

Paralytic ileus ____

Peristalsis ____

Peritonitis ____

Pyloric stenosis____

Rectus abdominis muscle ____

Salpingitis ____

Splenomegaly____

Striae ____

Umbilicus ____

COGNITIVE OBJECTIVES

At the end of this unit you will demonstrate knowledge of inspection, auscultation, percussion and palpation of the abdomen by your ability to:

1. Name the internal structures located in each of the quadrants of the abdomen.

2. Discuss normal findings associated with inspection of the skin, umbilicus, configuration, peristalsis and pulsations of the abdomen and name at least five common abdominal abnormalities which may be observed.

3. State the rationale for performing auscultation of the abdomen before percussion or palpation.

4. Describe the normal and abnormal sounds which may be heard in the abdomen.

5. Identify and give a rationale for the percussion notes heard over each quadrant of the abdomen. List at least four conditions which alter normal abdominal percussion notes.

6. Outline the procedure for percussing the borders of the liver and spleen.

7. Differentiate between light and deep palpation and state the purpose for each; name two common abnormalities which may be detected by light and deep palpation.

8. Discuss procedures for palpating characteristics of the liver, spleen, kidneys, masses and aortic pulsations.

9. State the method and rationale for determining the presence of costovertebral angle (CVA) and rebound tenderness.

10. Differentiate between visceral and parietal pain.

11. Describe common examination findings associated with appendicitis, pancreatitis, hernia, distended bladder, pregnant uterus, pyloric stenosis, ascites, abdominal tumor,

paralytic ileus, cirrhosis, cholecystitis, diverticulitis, malignancy, peritonitis, salpingitis, hepatitis, hepatomegaly, splenomegaly.

LEARNING ACTIVITIES

The Learning Activities contain information necessary for meeting the Cognitive Objectives. Select one and work with it until you have mastered the material. Use the Cognitive Objectives as a study guide. A Self-Test is provided so that you can check how much you know. If you have difficulty with the Self-Test, please review the material in this unit before proceeding to the Clinical Objectives.

Reading Activities

a) Bates: *A Guide to Physical Examination*, pp. 158–170. This section provides clear and concise coverage of relevant anatomy and physiology, step-by-step examination techniques with normal findings and illustrated tables of common abnormal findings. Numerous pictures and diagrams aid understanding.

b) DeGowin and DeGowin: *Bedside Diagnostic Examination*, pp. 452–530. This reading is geared to the more advanced practitioner and assumes familiarity with anatomy and physiology. It contains an in-depth coverage of examination techniques, abnormal findings and related key signs or symptoms of dysfunction.

c) Delp and Manning: *Major's Physical Diagnosis*, Chapter 9, "Examination of the Abdomen." Knowledge of anatomy and physiology of the abdomen is assumed. Examination findings and techniques are integrated in the text of the chapter. The emphasis is on differential diagnosis. The author has included a detailed table on abdominal distention. Supplement your learning with readings about the anatomical location of the abdominal organs and differential signs of visceral and parietal pain.

d) Gillies and Alyn: *Patient Assessment and Management by the Nurse Practitioner*, "Examination of the Abdomen" (pp. 86–100). This chapter presents comprehensive coverage of internal abdominal structures, procedures, techniques and normal examination findings. Some common abnormalities are included.

e) Judge and Zuidema: *Methods of Clinical Examination: A Physiologic Approach*, Chapter 11, "The Gastrointestinal System." This reading begins with a cursory discussion of examination procedures and normal findings, followed by cardinal symptoms and abnormal findings. You will need to supplement your learning with more detail as to procedures and findings. Use the Cognitive Objectives as a study guide.

f) Prior and Silberstein: *Physical Diagnosis*, Chapter 12, "The Abdomen." Reviews anatomy and physiology of the abdomen. Examination procedures are explained in detail. Emphasis is on normal findings. Visceral and somatic pain are well described. Contains informative photographs and diagrams.

g) Sana and Judge: *Physical Appraisal Methods in Nursing Practice*, Chapter 11, "Physical Appraisal of the Abdomen and the Male Genitourinary System." Assessment of the abdomen is presented clearly and systematically. Emphasis is on normal findings. This chapter includes a helpful glossary of terms and a review of the anatomical locations of the internal organs. Visceral and parietal pain are not covered. You may wish more detailed explanations of techniques and abnormalities.

h) Sherman and Fields: *Guide to Patient Evaluation*, pp. 154–168. This reading includes a cursory coverage of relevant anatomy and physiology. Examination techniques, normal features and basic abnormal findings are presented in an easy-to-follow manner. There is a sample recording of examination results using S.O.A.P., but this section does not include palpation of the abdominal aorta or differentiation between parietal and visceral pain.

Audiovisual Activity

a) Blue-Hill Educational Systems, Inc.: "The Abdomen." This video tape begins with a discussion of abdominal pain and then proceeds with the locations of abdominal contents in relation to anatomical landmarks. Physical examination techniques are described in detail. (The last part of the presentation covers evaluation of hernias and the rectal examination. This unit will cover only umbilical hernias.)

Supplemental Activities

The following materials are suggested to supplement or strengthen your learning.

a) Mansell, E. "Examination of the Abdomen." *AJN*, Sept. 1974. This programmed instruction presents anatomy and examination techniques for a basic abdominal examination.

b) A. H. Robins Co., Richmond, VA 23220: G. I. Series, "Physical Examination of the Abdomen" (I. Inspection, II. Palpation, III. Percussion, IV. Auscultation, V. Abdominal Pain, VI. Differential Diagnosis of Abdominal Disorders). This excellent series of booklets includes anatomy, physiology, techniques and findings as well as many illustrations.

SELF-TEST

This Self-Test is for you. Use it to check how well you have learned the material presented in this unit. The answers follow the test.

Match each of the following structures with the quadrant in which it is found.

1. _______ Appendix

2. _______ Left ovary

3. _______ Gallbladder

4. _______ Stomach

5. _______ Spleen

a) Right upper quadrant
b) Right lower quadrant
c) Left lower quadrant
d) Left upper quadrant

6. An abdomen which is bulging in appearance is described as
   a) protuberant.
   b) herniated.
   c) scaphoid.
   d) tympanic.

7. Separation of the rectus abdominis muscle most often occurs with
   1. obesity.
   2. inguinal hernia.
   3. pregnancy.
   4. surgical incision along the linea alba.
   5. splenomegaly.
   a) 3 only is correct.
   b) 2 only is correct.
   c) 1, 3 and 4 are correct.

    d) 2, 4 and 5 are correct.
    e) all of the above are correct.

8. Asymmetry of the abdomen occurs with
    1. obesity.
    2. ovarian tumor.
    3. pregnancy.
    4. gaseous distention.
    5. ascitic fluid.
    a) 2 only is correct.
    b) 2 and 3 are correct.
    c) 1, 4 and 5 are correct.
    d) 2 and 5 are correct.
    e) all of the above are correct.

9. Assessment of the abdomen includes noting
    1. location of scars.
    2. striae.
    3. rashes or lesions.
    4. venous pattern.
    5. bulging of the umbilicus.
    a) 3 and 5 are correct.
    b) 1, 2 and 4 are correct.
    c) 1, 3 and 5 are correct.
    d) 3, 4 and 5 are correct.
    e) all of the above are correct.

10. The umbilicus is normally assessed for
    a) contour and direction.
    b) color.
    c) hernia.
    d) a and c.
    e) all of the above.

11. While examining a client you observe strong abdominal pulsations between the xiphoid and umbilicus. When palpated, the pulsations expand laterally. You would suspect
    a) normal peristalsis.
    b) increased peristalsis due to early bowel obstruction.
    c) a mass overlying the aorta.
    d) an aortic aneurysm.
    e) borborygmi.

12. Auscultation of the abdomen is performed after inspection because
    a) other maneuvers tend to create augmented bowel sounds.
    b) auscultation usually follows inspection.
    c) percussion may be painful.
    d) palpation may alter placement of the organs and vessels.

13. Your client is 48 hours postoperative. After listening for 30 seconds at a site immediately below and to the right of the umbilicus, you do not hear any bowel sounds. Therefore, you decide that
    a) you are not listening in the right place.

    b)   the client has a partial bowel obstruction.
    c)   the client has gastritis.
    d)   you need to listen longer.

14. The normal percussion note(s) heard in the abdomen is (are)
        1.   resonance.
        2.   dullness.
        3.   tympany.
        4.   flatness.
        5.   hyperresonance.
    a)   1 only is correct.
    b)   2 and 5 are correct.
    c)   1, 2 and 3 are correct.
    d)   3 and 4 are correct.
    e)   all of the above are correct.

15. Percussion over the symphysis pubis in a client with a distended bladder would demonstrate a change in the percussion note from
    a)   resonant to hyperresonant.
    b)   tympanic to dull.
    c)   resonant to dull.
    d)   dull to resonant.
    e)   none of the above.

16. The procedure of percussing the liver borders for estimating its size includes
        1.   percussing downward from lung resonance in the left anterior axillary line.
        2.   percussing upward from the right lower quadrant along the right midclavicular line.
        3.   having the client exhale forcibly.
        4.   percussing downward from lung resonance to liver dullness in the midclavicular line.
    a)   2, 3 and 4 are correct.
    b)   1 and 2 are correct.
    c)   2 and 4 are correct.
    d)   1, 2 and 3 are correct.

17. Deep palpation is used to determine
        1.   organomegaly.
        2.   characteristics of masses.
        3.   relative density of internal structures.
        4.   tension of the abdominal musculature.
        5.   rebound tenderness.
    a)   1, 2 and 4 are correct.
    b)   1, 2 and 5 are correct.
    c)   1, 2 and 3 are correct.
    d)   4 and 5 are correct.
    e)   all of the above are correct.

18. Tenderness along the posterior costovertebral angles most often is indicative of
    a)   liver enlargement.
    b)   splenomegaly.
    c)   kidney infection.
    d)   ovarian cyst.
    e)   none of the above.

19. Visceral pain is usually
    1. sharp and well localized.
    2. dull and diffuse.
    3. referred.
    4. a manifestation of peritoneal involvement.
    5. due to stretching.
    a) 1 only is correct.
    b) 2 only is correct.
    c) 1, 3 and 4 are correct.
    d) 1, 2 and 4 are correct.
    e) 2 and 5 are correct.

SELF-TEST KEY

1. (b)

2. (c)

3. (a)

4. (d)

5. (d)

6. (a) Tympanic refers to a high-pitched percussion note as is heard over the gas-filled stomach bubble. Scaphoid describes a sunken abdomen or concave abdomen as found in severe malnutrition. Herniated describes an outpouching of structures through weak points in the abdominal wall. Protuberant means bulging or projecting.

7. (c) Diastasis recti occurs when the abdominal rectus muscles are separated by conditions which produce gross abdominal distention or surgical interruption along the midline (linea alba). Separation may also occur with epigastric or umbilical hernias. Enlargement of the spleen in the left upper quadrant is not usually sufficient to cause separation of the muscle.

8. (b) Generalized distention results from obesity, gas and ascites. Distention of the lower half of the abdomen or an asymmetrical distribution occurs with ovarian tumor, pregnancy or a distended bladder.

9. (e) Scars give pertinent information about the healing ability of the body as well as indicating previous trauma or surgery and alerting the examiner to the possibility of bowel obstruction or adhesions. Striae are multiple scars resulting from constant stretch of the skin (pregnancy, tumor, ascites). Rashes or lesions indicate primary or secondary problems (pruritus of obstructive jaundice). The venous pattern is normally very faint. In thin persons, the veins are more prominent. Obstruction of the vena cava or portal circulation causes engorgement of the veins. Bulging of the normally flat umbilicus may be caused by underlying masses, hernia or infection or ascites.

10. (e) Eversion or displacement from the normal position (midway between the xiphoid process and pubis) is a sign of hernia, fluid or masses. Discoloration of the

umbilical area occurs in various abnormal conditions and is due to blood pigments carried by the lymphatics.

11. (d) Peristalsis, if visible, occurs over the entire abdomen while aortic pulsations are primarily seen in the upper abdomen below the xiphoid. Normal peristalsis is increased with early bowel obstruction. Aortic pulsations are normally of low amplitude and are directed forward. A mass overlying the aorta will cause increased transmission of the pulsations. With an aneurysm of the abdominal aorta, the pulsations are transmitted laterally due to weakening of the vessel walls. Borborygmi is the term used to describe "stomach growling."

12. (a) Palpation and percussion stimulate artificial bowel sounds which will mask vascular sounds and give an incorrect assessment of the normal bowel sounds.

13. (d) Bowel sounds are heard over the entire abdomen but are usually heard best just below and to the right of the umbilicus. With partial bowel obstruction or gastritis, bowel sounds are increased. Normally bowel sounds occur 5 to 12 times per minute and are most frequent between meals and at night. However, postoperatively the bowel will be sluggish and you need to listen longer (5 minutes is recommended). Tapping the abdomen briskly will often stimulate peristalsis.

14. (c) Resonance is percussed over most of the abdomen, with areas of dullness over organs and tympany over the gastric air bubble. Flat percussion notes are heard over very dense substances (bone), and hyperresonance is characteristic of hyperinflation (emphysematous lung).

15. (c) The area over the symphysis pubis is normally resonant to percussion. When the bladder distends with urine, it rises up, above the pubis, presenting an area of greater density, which is percussed as dull.

16. (c) Percussion of the liver borders is performed along the right midclavicular line from lung resonance down to liver dullness and from below the level of the umbilicus upward to liver dullness. Extreme respiratory movements are not necessary for percussion.

17. (b) Deep palpation is used to assess location, shape, consistency, tenderness, pulsations and mobility of masses and to identify the size of organs and masses. Testing for rebound tenderness involves a deep probing motion. Estimating muscle tension or guarding is done by light palpation. Relative density is determined by percussion.

18. (c) Tenderness along the posterior costovertebral angles generally is an indication of kidney infection. Abnormalities of the liver and spleen may sometimes produce anterior costovertebral angle tenderness. The pain from ovarian cysts would most likely be unrelated to this maneuver.

19. (e) Visceral pain is due to stretching of the hollow viscus and is dull, aching and diffuse (menstrual cramps or gaseous distention). Parietal pain is caused by extension to the peritoneum. The pain is sharp and easily localized over the site or referred along the same dermatome as the pathological source (inflamed appendix, cholecystitis).

CLINICAL COMPONENT

Having completed the cognitive portion of this unit, you are now ready to proceed to the Clinical Objectives. The purpose of the Clinical Component is to help you learn to assess the abdomen for normal configuration and organ function and to detect the presence, location and extent of any dysfunction.

CLINICAL OBJECTIVES

At the end of this unit you will perform systematic assessment of the abdomen, correlating physical examination skills with physiological principles. You will be able to:

1. Demonstrate knowledge of signs and symptoms of dysfunction related to the abdomen by obtaining a pertinent health history from the client.

2. Demonstrate inspection of the abdomen by assessing configuration, skin, umbilicus, peristalsis and pulsations.

3. Demonstrate auscultation of the abdomen by assessing characteristics of bowel sounds and presence of bruits.

4. Demonstrate percussion of the abdomen by
    a. identifying the distribution of tympany and dullness in the abdomen.
    b. outlining the borders of the liver and spleen.

5. Demonstrate light palpation by assessing superficial organs, masses, muscular resistance and tenderness.

6. Demonstrate deep palpation by assessing
    a. the contour of the liver, spleen and kidneys.
    b. masses for location, shape, consistency, tenderness and mobility.
    c. presence of costovertebral angle or rebound tenderness.
    d. aortic pulsations.

7. Utilize S.O.A.P. to systematically describe findings, make an assessment regarding normality and formulate a plan of action.

INSTRUCTIONS

Utilizing three of your peers or clients in the clinical area, practice inspection, auscultation, percussion and palpation of the abdomen. Remove the Performance Guide cards for Unit 21 from Appendix II. These cards will enable you to practice the skills necessary to meet the Clinical Objectives and complete the Response Sheets. On each Response Sheet you will be expected to (1) ask questions which elicit possible symptoms, (2) systematically describe your findings, (3) localize any abnormalities present and (4) summarize your examination findings using the S.O.A.P. method of recording.

When you have mastered the Clinical Objectives and completed the Response Sheets, arrange to demonstrate your skills to your laboratory instructor or preceptor.

EQUIPMENT

Stethoscope
Tangential lighting
Tape measure
Warm hands

OPTIONAL ACTIVITIES

These activities demonstrate techniques of abdominal assessment.
a)   Bates: "The Abdomen" (film).
b)   Blue-Hill Educational Systems, Inc.: "The Abdomen," a video tape cassette (35 minutes).

RESPONSE SHEET—ABDOMINAL EXAMINATION

Client ___________________________

Date _________________ Age _______ Sex _______

Examiner ___________________________

I. Health History

II. Inspection

    A. Position

    B. Contour, Symmetry

    C. Skin

    D. Umbilicus

    E. Movements

III. Auscultation

    A. Bowel Sounds

    B. Circulatory Sounds

IV. Light Palpation

    A. Muscular Tension

B. Enlarged Organs

C. Masses

V. Deep Palpation

A. Masses

B. Rebound/CVA Tenderness

C. Liver

D. Spleen

E. Kidneys

F. Aorta

VI. Percussion

A. Gas Pattern/General Areas of Dullness

B. Liver

C. Spleen

D. Bladder

E. Fluid

Summarize your findings using the S.O.A.P. method.

S. **(Client's observations, complaints, health history)**

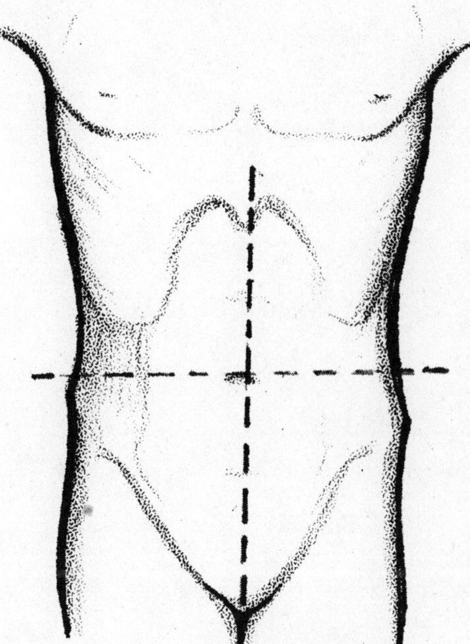

O. **(Physical findings)**

A. **(Assessment of the problem, data, prognosis)**

P. **(Plans for further evaluation, care, treatment)**

RESPONSE SHEET—ABDOMINAL EXAMINATION

Client _______________________________________

Date _______________________ Age _______ Sex _______

Examiner _______________________________________

I. Health History

II. Inspection

    A. Position

    B. Contour, Symmetry

    C. Skin

    D. Umbilicus

    E. Movements

III. Auscultation

    A. Bowel Sounds

    B. Circulatory Sounds

IV. Light Palpation

    A. Muscular Tension

    B. Enlarged Organs

    C. Masses

V. Deep Palpation

    A. Masses

    B. Rebound/CVA Tenderness

    C. Liver

    D. Spleen

    E. Kidneys

    F. Aorta

VI. Percussion

    A. Gas Pattern/General Areas of Dullness

    B. Liver

    C. Spleen

    D. Bladder

    E. Fluid

Summarize your findings using the S.O.A.P. method.

S. (Client's observations, complaints, health history)

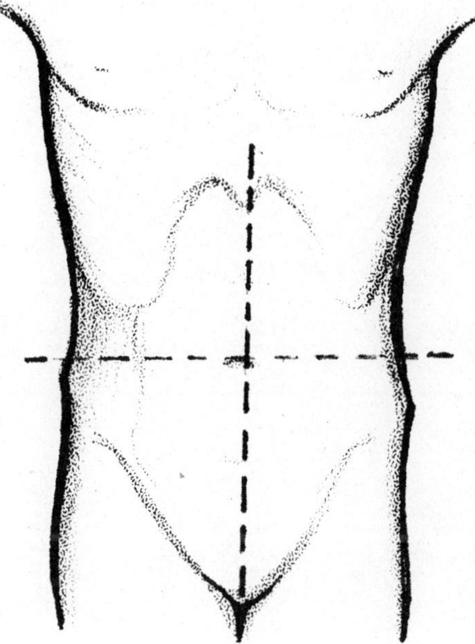

O. (Physical findings)

A. (Assessment of the problem, data, prognosis)

P. (Plans for further evaluation, care, treatment)

Client ________________________________

Date ___________________ Age _______ Sex _______

Examiner ______________________________

I. **Health History**

II. **Inspection**

    A. **Position**

    B. **Contour, Symmetry**

    C. **Skin**

    D. **Umbilicus**

    E. **Movements**

III. **Auscultation**

    A. **Bowel Sounds**

    B. **Circulatory Sounds**

IV. **Light Palpation**

    A. **Muscular Tension**

    B. Enlarged Organs

    C. Masses

V. Deep Palpation

    A. Masses

    B. Rebound/CVA Tenderness

    C. Liver

    D. Spleen

    E. Kidneys

    F. Aorta

VI. Percussion

    A. Gas Pattern/General Areas of Dullness

    B. Liver

    C. Spleen

    D. Bladder

    E. Fluid

Summarize your findings using the S.O.A.P. method.

S. (Client's observations, complaints, health history)

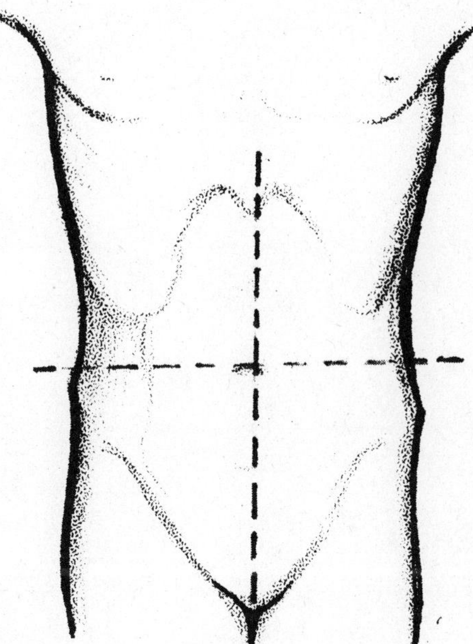

O. (Physical findings)

A. (Assessment of the problem, data, prognosis)

P. (Plans for further evaluation, care, treatment)

UNIT 22

Identify the following structures in the accompanying illustration.

1. _______ Prostate

2. _______ Testis

3. _______ Glans

4. _______ Vas deferens

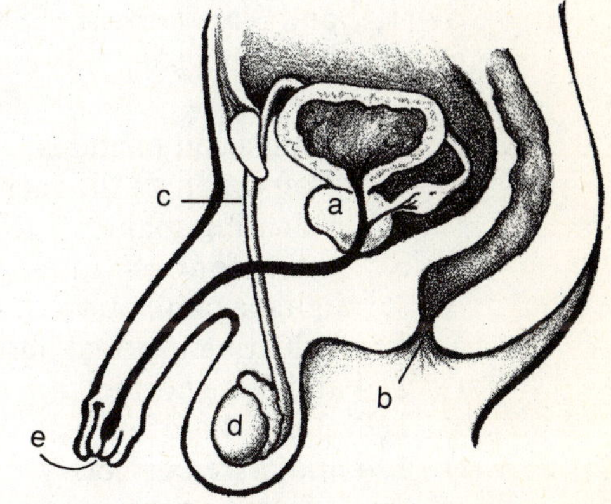

5. Enlargement of the prostate
    1. commonly occurs in men over age 50.
    2. frequently occurs with prostatitis.
    3. causes varying degrees of urinary tract impairment.
    4. is always a sign of malignancy.
  a) 1 and 3 are correct.
  b) 2 and 4 are correct.
  c) 1, 2 and 3 are correct.
  d) all of the above are correct.

6. A slit-like tear in the superficial anal mucosa is called
  a) pilonidal cyst.
  b) anal fissure.
  c) rectal tag.
  d) anorectal fistula.

7. Examination of the penis includes
    1. retraction of the foreskin to inspect the glans.
    2. noting the location of the urethral meatus.
    3. palpating the shaft for induration, nodules.
    4. describing size, shape, skin color, lesions, nodules.
    5. noting hygiene and characteristics of discharge if present.
  a) 1 and 2 are correct.
  b) 2, 3 and 4 are correct.
  c) 3, 4 and 5 are correct.
  d) all of the above are correct.

8. The following statements concern preparation for genitourinary and rectal examination.
    1. Inform the client of purpose and steps in the procedure after the examination.
    2. Have all equipment within easy reach: gloves, lubricant, movable exam light.
    3. The examiner must have short fingernails.
    4. Men are less modest than women, so draping is not essential.
    5. Administer a cleansing enema prior to examination.
   a) 1, 2, 3 and 5 are correct.
   b) 2 and 3 are correct.
   c) 1, 2 and 4 are correct.
   d) 1, 2 and 3 are correct.
   e) all of the above are correct.

9. Rectal examination includes
    1. observation of the sacrococcygeal and perianal areas.
    2. evaluating sphincter tone.
    3. testing for occult blood.
    4. digital examination of the prostate.
    5. evaluating inguinal hernias if present.
   a) 2, 4 and 5 are correct.
   b) 1, 2, 3 and 4 are correct.
   c) 1, 4 and 5 are correct.
   d) 3 and 5 are correct.
   e) all of the above are correct.

10. On examination you note that the testes are small and soft. This is probably due to
   a) virilism.
   b) torsion.
   c) atrophy associated with aging.
   d) cryptorchidism.
   e) normal response to warm external temperatures.

11. During inspection and palpation of the scrotum, you should
    1. check for skin color, lesions, nodules.
    2. note size and contour.
    3. identify the characteristics of the testes and epididymides.
    4. palpate along the spermatic cord.
    5. assess inguinal hernias.
   a) 1 and 2 are correct.
   b) 1, 2, 3 and 4 are correct.
   c) 1, 2, 3 and 5 are correct.
   d) 3, 4 and 5 are correct.
   e) all of the above are correct.

12. Placement of the urethral meatus on the ventral surface of the penis is
    1. normal.
    2. a congenital anomaly.
    3. epispadias.
    4. phimosis.
    5. a possible cause of psychological problems.
   a) 2 and 5 are correct.
   b) 1 only is correct.

    c) 2, 3 and 5 are correct.
    d) 4 only is correct.
    e) 4 and 5 are correct.

13. Mr. Johnson complains of scrotal pain. Examination reveals the left epididymis and vas deferens to be swollen and tender. You suspect
    a) scrotal hernia.
    b) tumor.
    c) epididymitis.
    d) varicocele.
    e) syphilis.

14. In transillumination of the scrotum
    1. the scrotal contents are identified.
    2. most scrotal contents are opaque.
    3. structures containing blood or tissue are opaque.
    4. structures containing serous fluid transilluminate easily.
    5. the epididymis transilluminates.
    a) 1, 3, 4 and 5 are correct.
    b) 1, 2, 3 and 4 are correct.
    c) 1, 2 and 5 are correct.
    d) 3 and 4 are correct.
    e) all of the above are correct.

15. Scrotal edema presents with
    1. nephrosis.
    2. cardiac decompensation.
    3. thrombosis of the pelvic veins.
    4. portal vein obstruction.
    5. blockage of the inguinal lymphatics.
    a) 3, 4 and 5 are correct.
    b) 1 and 2 are correct.
    c) 1, 3 and 4 are correct.
    d) 1, 2 and 5 are correct.
    e) all of the above are correct.

16. The scrotum contains
    a) epididymides, testes, and vas deferens.
    b) testes, epididymides, vas deferens, blood vessels and nerves.
    c) spermatic cords and testes.
    d) prostate, vas deferens and testes.

17. Mr. Alexander complains of a growth on his penis. Inspection and palpation reveal a nontender nodule with an indurated base located on the shaft near the glans. This is most likely
    a) herpes genitalias.
    b) gonorrhea.
    c) syphilis.
    d) carcinoma.
    e) chancroid.

18. The following statements refer to characteristics of hernias.
    1. The most common type of hernia in the groin is an indirect inguinal hernia.

    2. An indirect inguinal hernia appears at the midline of the inguinal ligament, near the internal inguinal ring.

    3. A direct inguinal hernia is usually found near the external inguinal ring near the pubis.

    4. Femoral hernias occur below the inguinal ligament, medial to the femoral artery.

    5. Direct inguinal hernias most often progress into the scrotum.

a) 1, 2, 4 and 5 are correct.
b) 1, 2, 3 and 4 are correct.
c) 2 and 4 are correct.
d) all of the above are correct.
e) none of the above are correct.

19. The normal prostate gland is palpated

    1. only on the anterior surface.
    2. as a rounded structure with two symmetrical lobes.
    3. as having a very hard and nodular surface.
    4. as approximately 2.5 cm long.
    5. as being softer and smaller in older men.

a) 2 and 4 are correct.
b) 1, 2, 3 and 4 are correct.
c) 2 only is correct.
d) 1, 3 and 5 are correct.
e) 1 and 4 are correct.

20. Mr. Phelps' chief complaint is an enlarged, nontender scrotum of one week's duration. Examination of the scrotum reveals a mass within the tunica vaginalis that transilluminates readily. You suspect

a) scrotal hernia.
b) varicocele.
c) hydrocele.
d) carcinoma.
e) gonorrheal orchitis.

Number 22

The Genitourinary and Rectal Examination (Male)

RATIONALE

This self-instructional unit is designed to help you learn inspection and palpation of the male genitalia and related areas. The primary emphasis is on systematic assessment of the genitalia and inguinal and rectal areas and description of normal findings. Common abnormalities will also be discussed.

GLOSSARY OF TERMS

Review the following terms before and after completing this unit. You should be able to define or describe them readily.

Benign prostatic hypertrophy (BPH) ____

Chancre ____

Chancroid ____

Condyloma acuminatum ____

Cryptorchidism ____

Cystitis ____

Epididymis ____

Epispadias ____

Hemorrhoid ____

Hernia ____

Herpes genitalis ____

Hydrocele ____

Hypospadias ____

Infantilism ____

Orchitis ____

Peyronie's disease ____

Phimosis ____

Prepuce ____

Priapism ____

Smegma ____

Spermatic cord ____

Spermatocele ____

Torsion ____

Varicocele ____

Vas deferens ____

OGNITIVE OBJECTIVES

At the end of this unit you will demonstrate knowledge of inspection and palpation of the ale genitalia and inguinal and rectal areas by your ability to:

1. Identify on a drawing or model the following external and internal structures:
   a. Penile shaft, prepuce, glans, corona, urethral meatus, scrotum, anus.
   b. Symphysis pubis, bladder, rectum, vas deferens, spermatic cord, urethra, epididymis, testes, prostate gland, external and internal inguinal rings.

2. Discuss preparation of the client and psychosocial aspects of the genitourinary and rectal examination.

3. Describe the examination procedure and normal findings for inspection and palpation of the penis and scrotum; discuss transillumination.

4. Outline the procedure for evaluation of hernias; differentiate between femoral, direct and indirect inguinal hernias; discuss causative factors and implications related to disorders.

5. Describe techniques and normal findings for the rectal examination: sacrococcygeal and perianal areas, anus and prostate gland.

6. Describe causative factors and examination findings associated with abnormalities.
   a. Groin: hernias, enlarged lymph glands.
   b. Penis: hypospadias, epispadias, condyloma acuminatum, Peyronie's disease, infantilism, virilism, phimosis, carcinoma, priapism, urethritis, cystitis.

   c. Scrotum: hydrocele, scrotal hernia, testicular torsion, tumor, spermatocele, epididymitis, varicocele, sebaceous cyst, orchitis, atrophy, edema, cryptorchidism.

   d. Anus and rectum: polyps, hemorrhoids, anorectal fistula, pilonidal cyst, pruritus ani, anal fissure.

   e. Prostate: benign prostatic hypertrophy (BPH), prostatitis.

7. Discuss signs and symptoms of common venereal diseases, examination precautions and psychosocial aspects: syphilis, gonorrhea, chancroid, herpes genitalis, granuloma inguinale.

LEARNING ACTIVITIES

The Learning Activities contain information necessary for meeting the Cognitive Objectives. Select one and proceed to work with it until you have mastered the material. Use the Cognitive Objectives as a study guide. A Self-Test is provided so that you can check how much you know. If you have difficulty with the Self-Test, please review the material in this unit before proceeding to the Clinical Objectives.

Reading Activities

a) Bates: *A Guide to Physical Examination*, Chapter 10, "Male Genitalia and Hernias," pp. 179–187. This chapter includes a comprehensive review of anatomy and physiology of the male genitalia, step-by-step instruction for examination, and tables of common abnormal findings. Excellent illustrations aid in learning. Assessment of the anus and rectum is presented in a separate chapter.

b) DeGowin and DeGowin: *Bedside Diagnostic Examination*, Chapter 9, "The Genitalia." This source is useful for the practitioner desiring extensive information. Anatomy, physiology and examination techniques are presented in detail, but the information is scattered throughout the text. Emphasis is on differentiating abnormalities.

c) Delp and Manning: *Major's Physical Diagnosis*, Chapter 13. Knowledge of anatomy and physiology is assumed. This chapter describes general examination techniques and common abnormal findings for the inguinal area, genitalia and rectal area and contains informative photographs of abnormalities. Psychological aspects are stressed throughout.

d) Gillies and Alyn: *Patient Assessment and Management by the Nurse Practitioner*, pp. 100–102. Knowledge of anatomy and physiology is assumed. This section includes information about examination of the male genitalia and rectum. Psychosocial aspects and hernias are not covered. Supplement your reading as necessary to learn about the abnormalities listed in the Cognitive Objectives.

e) Judge and Zuidema: *Methods of Clinical Examination: A Physiologic Approach*, Chapter 14, "Genitourinary System," pp. 241–253. Knowledge of anatomy and physiology is assumed. An overview of the examination and normal findings is followed by discussion of cardinal symptoms and abnormal findings. Supplement learning in all areas.

f) Prior and Silberstein: *Physical Diagnosis,* Chapter 13, "Genitalia," pp. 306–312. Knowledge of anatomy is assumed. Examination procedures, normal findings and common abnormal findings are well covered. Refer to Chapter 12 for information on hernias and rectal examination. You may wish to supplement your learning with readings which describe procedural techniques in more detail.

g) Sana and Judge: *Physical Appraisal Methods in Nursing Practice*, Chapter 11, "Physical Appraisal of the Abdomen and the Male Genitourinary System," pp. 221–227. Knowledge of anatomy is assumed. Procedures and normal findings are briefly covered. Evaluation of inguinal hernias is well presented. Supplement learning in all areas to meet the Cognitive Objectives.

h) Sherman and Fields: *Guide to Patient Evaluation*. In this overview of anatomy and physiology, examination procedures are easy to follow and normal findings are emphasized. Supplementation will be necessary.

Audiovisual Activity

a) Blue-Hill Educational Systems, Inc.: "The Genitourologic Examination (Male)." This 30-minute video tape cassette reviews pertinent anatomy and physiology. Systematic assessment is stressed, with emphasis on technique and normal findings. Abnormal findings are presented in detail. The last part of "Abdominal Examination" should also be viewed for material on hernias and the rectal examination (approximately 15 minutes).

Supplemental Activity

The following material is suggested to strengthen your learning.
a) Eli Lilly and Co.: "Venereal Lesions in the Male," 28 color slides of venereal lesions.

SELF-TEST

This Self-Test is for you. Use it to check how well you have learned the material presented in the unit. The answers follow the test.

1. Identify the internal and external structures labeled on the following illustration.

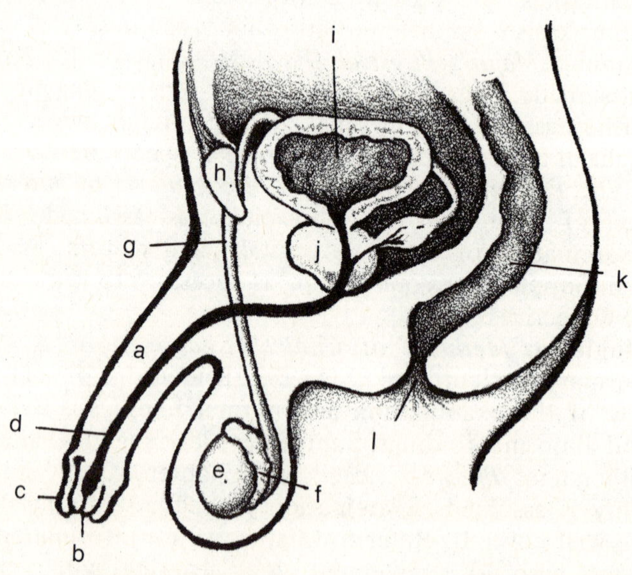

a) _______________________   g) _______________________

b) _______________________   h) _______________________

c) _______________________   i) _______________________

d) _______________________   j) _______________________

e) _______________________   k) _______________________

f) _______________________   l) _______________________

2. Symptoms which should alert the examiner to dysfunction include
    1. recent appearance of a "pimple" on the penis.
    2. enlargement of the scrotum.
    3. rectal bleeding.
    4. difficulty starting a urinary stream.
    5. small genitalia.
  a) 1 and 3 are correct.
  b) 2 and 4 are correct.
  c) 1, 2, 3 and 4 are correct.
  d) all of the above are correct.

3. In the preparation of a male client for a genitourinary and rectal examination,
    1. inform him of the steps in the procedure before performing them.
    2. have all equipment within reach.
    3. it is mandatory for the examiner to have short fingernails.
    4. the drape can be omitted since men are less modest than women.
    5. the client is instructed to use a laxative or cleansing enema the night before.
  a) 1, 2, 3 and 5 are correct.
  b) 2, 3 and 5 are correct.
  c) 1, 2 and 3 are correct.
  d) 1, 2 and 4 are correct.
  e) all of the above are correct.

4. In the examination of the penis
    1. note size and contour.
    2. inspect the skin for inflammation, lesions and nodules.
    3. retract the foreskin to inspect the prepuce.
    4. note location of urethral meatus and characteristics of discharge if present.
    5. palpate the shaft for nodules and induration.
  a) all of the above are correct.
  b) 1, 2 and 4 are correct.
  c) 2, 4 and 5 are correct.
  d) all of the above are correct.

5. _______________is the condition in which the prepuce cannot be retracted.

6. The urethral meatus is normally located on the_______________of the glans and is the

    opening through which _______________is (are) released.

7. List the contents of the scrotum.

____

____

8. Inspection and palpation of the scrotum includes
    1. checking skin color, lesions, nodules.
    2. noting size and contour.
    3. identifying the characteristics of the testes and epididymides.
    4. palpating along the length of the spermatic cord.
    5. evaluating the characteristics of the prostate gland.
   a) 2, 3 and 5 are correct.
   b) 1, 2, 3 and 4 are correct.
   c) 1, 3, 4 and 5 are correct.
   d) all of the above are correct.

9. In transillumination of the scrotum
    1. the scrotal contents are evaluated.
    2. most scrotal contents transilluminate.
    3. structures containing blood or tissue are opaque.
    4. structures containing serous fluid transilluminate.
   a) 2 and 4 are correct.
   b) 1, 3 and 4 are correct.
   c) 1 and 2 are correct.
   d) all of the above are correct.
   e) none of the above are correct.

10. Asymmetry of the scrotal sac in which one side is smaller is found with
    1. normal variant.
    2. atrophy.
    3. testis and epididymis absent.
    4. cryptorchidism.
    5. retraction into the inguinal canal.
   a) 1 only is correct.
   b) 3 and 5 are correct.
   c) 2 and 4 are correct.
   d) all of the above are correct.

11. Enlargement of the scrotal contents is found with
    1. hydrocele.
    2. testicular tumor.
    3. spermatocele.
    4. epididymitis.
    5. varicocele.
   a) all of the above are correct.
   b) none of the above are correct.
   c) 1, 3 and 4 are correct.
   d) 2, 4 and 5 are correct.

12. Scrotal edema occurs with
    1. congestive heart failure.
    2. nephrosis.
    3. portal vein obstruction.
    4. thrombosis of the pelvic veins.
    5. blockage of inguinal lymphatics.
   a) 3, 4 and 5 are correct.
   b) 1, 3 and 4 are correct.

   c)   2 and 5 are correct.
   d)   none of the above are correct.
   e)   all of the above are correct.

13.   Conditions which cause acute testicular pain include
      1.   gonorrheal orchitis.
      2.   torsion of the spermatic cord.
      3.   large hydrocele.
      4.   epididymitis.
      5.   sebaceous cyst.
   a)   1, 2 and 4 are correct.
   b)   3 and 5 are correct.
   c)   1, 2, 3 and 4 are correct.
   d)   all of the above are correct.

14.   Rectal examination includes
      1.   observation of the sacrococcygeal and perianal areas.
      2.   evaluation of sphincter tone.
      3.   testing for occult blood.
      4.   digital examination of the prostate.
      5.   evaluation of femoral hernias and rectal masses.
   a)   2, 4 and 5 are correct.
   b)   1, 2, 3 and 4 are correct.
   c)   1, 4 and 5 are correct.
   d)   3 and 5 are correct.
   e)   all of the above are correct.

15.   An opening between the rectum and the skin surface is known as ______________

      _____________.

16.   Only the_______________ surface of the prostate gland can be palpated. It has

      __________lobes and is approximately__________cm long.

17.   In an examination for hernias,
      1.   ask the client to lift a heavy object and note any bulging in the inguinal or femoral area.
      2.   the supine position is best for evaluating hernias.
      3.   ask the client to strain or bear down and note any suspicious bulges in the groin.
      4.   rectal examination will aid in differentiating direct and indirect hernias.
   a)   1, 2 and 3 are correct.
   b)   3 only is correct.
   c)   2 and 4 are correct.
   d)   1 and 4 are correct.
   e)   all of the above are correct.

18.   When venereal disease is suspected, the examiner should remember
      1.   to maintain a nonjudgmental attitude.
      2.   that gloves are not necessary unless there is a break in the skin.
      3.   that it is necessary to treat only the client and not his partner.
      4.   that VD is most prevalent in the lower socioeconomic classes.

a) 1 only is correct.
b) 2, 3 and 4 are correct.
c) 1, 3 and 4 are correct.
d) 1, 2 and 3 are correct.
e) all of the above are correct.

SELF-TEST KEY

1. (a) penile shaft
   (b) glans
   (c) prepuce
   (d) urethra
   (e) testis
   (f) epididymis
   (g) vas deferens
   (h) symphysis pubis
   (i) bladder
   (j) prostate gland
   (k) rectum
   (l) anus

2. (d) The complaint of a "pimple" may indicate anything from an infected hair follicle to venereal disease. Scrotal enlargement can reflect trauma, hernia, infection or a growth. Edema of the scrotum may be secondary to generalized edema. Rectal bleeding is a frequent complaint with hemorrhoids and constipation but may indicate more serious conditions. Be sure to determine the exact amount of bleeding. Difficulty with urination is frequently associated with enlargement of the prostate (BPH) in older men. However, it may also indicate infection, mechanical obstruction or neurological dysfunction. Abnormally small genitalia may be caused by endocrine imbalance (infantilism) or may be the result of trauma (testicular atrophy). Undue preoccupation with genital size requires respect for the client's concern but in some cases may indicate a need for psychological evaluation.

3. (c) Examination of the sexual organs has a personal and emotional significance not reserved for women alone. A drape is cumbersome if the client is examined in a sitting or standing position. However, in specific situations an appropriate drape should be used. It is important for the examiner to demonstrate professional and personal respect for the client's covert or overt concerns. Brief explanations beforehand of the purpose and steps in the examining procedure will help to allay apprehension.

   Having your equipment at hand is an important part of any procedure and prevents unnecessary delay or fumbling which might add to the client's apprehension. Adequate palpation cannot be performed with long fingernails without causing a great deal of discomfort.

   Under normal conditions, the rectum should not be cleansed prior to examination, since this may distort findings. Additionally, the small amount of stool which adheres to the examiner's glove can be tested for occult blood.

4. (d) Assessment of the penis includes noting the size, shape and characteristics of the skin. If present, the foreskin (prepuce) is retracted to inspect the glans, placement of the urethral meatus and presence of discharge. Purulent discharge should be checked for gonorrhea. The shaft is palpated for any nodules or induration.

5. Phimosis is the condition in which the foreskin or prepuce cannot be retracted. Paraphimosis refers to the condition in which the prepuce has been retracted and then cannot be drawn forward over the glans.

6. Tip; urine and semen. The urethral opening is located at the tip of the glans. In congenital conditions it may be located on the ventral surface (hypospadias) or dorsal

surface (epispadias). Both urine and semen are released through the same orifice in the male.

7. Testes, epididymides, spermatic cords, vas deferens, blood and lymph vessels, nerves and muscle fibers are the contents of the scrotum.

8. (b) The walls of the scrotum are examined for size, contour, color, lesions and nodules. The testes and epididymides are identified and palpated for size, contour and tenderness. The spermatic cord is identified and palpated from the external inguinal ring to the testis. Examination of the prostate is not possible via the scrotum.

9. (b) Transillumination is the process of shining a light from behind the scrotum in order to better visualize the contents. Structures containing tissue or blood (normal contents, masses, hernias, hematoceles) are opaque. Structures containing serous fluid allow the light to pass through (hydrocele).

10. (d) Asymmetry of the scrotum is a normal occurrence, with the right side usually smaller than the left (the spermatic cord is longer on the left). Atrophy, absence, retraction or failure of a testis to descend are all cases in which one side of the scrotum may appear to be smaller than the other.

11. (a) Masses such as found with hydrocele, spermatocele and tumor are palpated as enlargements within the sac. Inflammation of the epididymis results in tenderness and swelling. Varicocele (varicosities of the spermatic cord) is felt as a soft mass or "bag of worms."

12. (e) Because of the scrotum's dependent position and proximity to the peritoneal cavity, scrotal edema results when there is generalized edema (cardiac decompensation), altered pressure gradients (nephrosis) or portal vein obstruction. Blockage of the pelvic veins or inguinal lymph vessels also results in scrotal edema.

13. (c) Acute testicular pain occurs with infection (gonorrhea, epididymitis), trauma (hematoma, torsion of the cord, incarcerated scrotal hernia) and pressure on the testis due to development of a large hydrocele within the tunica vaginalis. Sebaceous cysts usually develop on the outside of the scrotal wall and are nontender.

14. (b) Observation of the skin in the rectal area is important for evaluating cysts, fissures, skin irritation and lesions. The tone of the rectal sphincter is evaluated during digital examination. While practitioners do not always test for occult blood, it is a simple matter to test the stool which adheres to the examining glove. Many texts encourage routine testing for occult blood. Assessing the size, contour and consistency of the prostate gland is an important part of rectal examination in the male. Femoral hernias cannot be evaluated rectally. The characteristics of any rectal masses should be noted.

15. Anorectal fistula. An anorectal fistula results from an inflammatory tract which drains from the anus or rectum out to the external skin. Do not confuse the terminology with anal fissure, which is an ulceration of the anal mucosa.

16. Only the posterior surface of the prostate gland can be palpated. It has 2 lobes and is 2.5 cm long.

17. (b) If a hernia is suspected, the upright position will best demonstrate its appearance because of the weight of the abdominal organs on the weakened muscle wall. As the

client strains or bears down, the additional pressure will cause the hernia bulge to become more apparent. Asking the client to lift a heavy object will have a similar effect but runs the risk of causing further injury! Palpation of the scrotum and inguinal canal will help to differentiate between direct and indirect inguinal hernias.

18. (a) VD is not limited by social or economic status. It is the responsibility of the examiner to maintain an objective and caring attitude in order to promote the trustworthy relationship necessary for planning treatment of VD. Unless a client's sexual partners are treated, infection will recur. Gloves are always recommended when examining lesions or suspect conditions, as a break in the skin is not necessary for infection by some organisms to occur!

CLINICAL COMPONENT

Having completed the cognitive portion of this unit, you are now ready to proceed to the Clinical Objectives. The purpose of the Clinical Component is to assess the male genitourinary system and rectum for normal configuration and function and to detect the presence, location and extent of any dysfunction.

CLINICAL OBJECTIVES

At the end of this unit you will perform a genitourinary and rectal examination of the male, correlating physical assessment skills with physiological principles. You will be able to:

1. Demonstrate knowledge of signs and symptoms related to dysfunction by obtaining a pertinent health history from the client.

2. Demonstrate knowledge of psychosocial factors related to examination of the sexual organs by appropriate preparation of the client and interaction throughout the procedure.

3. Demonstrate systematic inspection and palpation for general characteristics of the penis, scrotum, groin, anus and rectum.

4. Demonstrate palpation of the scrotum by identifying the characteristics of the testes, epididymides and spermatic cords; demonstrate transillumination.

5. Demonstrate palpation for hernias.

6. Demonstrate rectal examination, noting sphincter tone and characteristics of the prostate gland.

7. Utilize the S.O.A.P. method of recording to systematically describe findings, make an assessment regarding normality and formulate a plan of action.

INSTRUCTIONS

Utilizing three of your peers or clients in the clinical area, practice inspection and palpation of the male genitourinary and rectal system. Remove the Performance Guide cards for Unit 22 from Appendix II. These cards will enable you to practice the skills necessary to meet the Clinical Objectives and complete the Response Sheets. On each Response Sheet you will be expected to (1) ask questions which elicit possible symptoms, (2) systematically describe your findings, (3) localize any abnormalities present and (4) summarize your examination findings using the S.O.A.P. method of recording.

When you have mastered the Clinical Objectives and completed the Response Sheets, arrange to demonstrate your skills to your laboratory instructor or preceptor.

EQUIPMENT

Drape
Gloves
Lubricant and paper towel
Materials for testing for occult blood
Materials for collecting other specimens (optional)
Examination table
Movable stool
Gooseneck lamp or other light
Penlight (small flashlight)
Tissues

OPTIONAL ACTIVITIES

These activities demonstrate techniques for assessment of the male genitourinary and rectal systems.

a) Bates: "The Male Genitalia, Anus and Rectum" (film).

b) Blue-Hill Educational Systems, Inc.: "Genitourologic" (a 12-minute video tape cassette).

RESPONSE SHEET—GENITOURINARY AND RECTAL EXAMINATION (MALE)

Client _______________________________

Date _________________ Age _______________

Examiner _______________________________

I. Health History

II. Physical Examination

   A. Penis

      1. Shaft

      2. Prepuce

      3. Glans

   B. Scrotum

      1. General

      2. Testes

      3. Epididymides

   C. Groin

D. Rectal Area

1. Skin

2. Anus

3. Rectum

4. Prostate

5. Occult blood

Summarize your findings using the S.O.A.P. method.

S. **(Client's observations, complaints, health history)**

O. **(Physical findings)**

A. **(Assessment of the problem, data, prognosis)**

P. **(Plans for further evaluation, care, teaching)**

RESPONSE SHEET—GENITOURINARY AND RECTAL EXAMINATION (MALE)

Client ____

Date _______________________ Age _______________

Examiner ____

I. Health History

II. Physical Examination

A. Penis

1. Shaft

2. Prepuce

3. Glans

B. Scrotum

1. General

2. Testes

3. Epididymides

C. Groin

D. Rectal Area

1. Skin

2. Anus

3. Rectum

4. Prostate

5. Occult blood

Summarize your findings using the S.O.A.P. method.

S. (Client's observations, complaints, health history)

O. (Physical findings)

A. (Assessment of the problem, data, prognosis)

P. (Plans for further evaluation, care, teaching)

RESPONSE SHEET—GENITOURINARY AND RECTAL EXAMINATION (MALE)

Client _______________________________

Date _________________ Age _____________

Examiner _____________________________

I. **Health History**

II. **Physical Examination**

   A. **Penis**

      1. Shaft

      2. Prepuce

      3. Glans

   B. **Scrotum**

      1. General

      2. Testes

      3. Epididymides

   C. **Groin**

D. Rectal Area

1. Skin

2. Anus

3. Rectum

4. Prostate

5. Occult blood

Summarize your findings using the S.O.A.P. method.

S. (Client's observations, complaints, health history)

O. (Physical findings)

A. (Assessment of the problem, data, prognosis)

P. (Plans for further evaluation, care, teaching)

PRE-TEST

UNIT 23

Identify the following anatomical structures in the accompanying illustration:

1. _______ Bladder

2. _______ Uterus

3. _______ Ovary

4. _______ Vagina

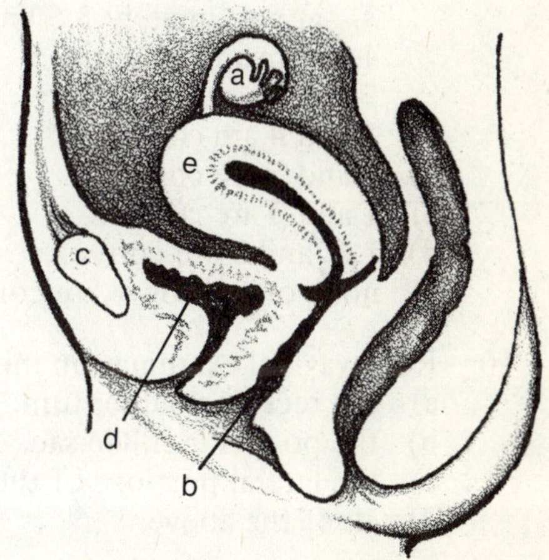

5. In regard to Bartholin's glands,
   a) the openings are located below and to either side of the urethral meatus.
   b) infection may result in labial swelling.
   c) normally they are palpable.
   d) statements in b and c are correct.
   e) all of the above statements are correct.

6. The adnexal areas
   a) are palpated for shape, size, consistency and mobility of masses.
   b) are examined for symmetry and tenderness.
   c) include the ovaries, fallopian tubes and supporting ligaments.
   d) are described in both b and c.
   e) are described by all of the above.

7. The vaginal mucosa in adult women is normally
   a) pale, pink and dry.
   b) bluish.
   c) red and moist.
   d) pink and slightly moist.
   e) none of the above.

8. The cervix is
   1. normally firm, smooth and mobile.
   2. normally hard, smooth and immobile.
   3. tender when palpated.

    4. nontender when palpated.

    5. softer than normal during pregnancy.

a) 1 and 3 are correct.

b) 2 and 3 are correct.

c) 1, 4 and 5 are correct.

d) 2, 4 and 5 are correct.

e) 2 and 4 are correct.

9. During bimanual palpation the uterus is normally felt to be

    1. spongy.

    2. rigidly fixed.

    3. approximately 3.5 cm long.

    4. firm and smooth.

    5. nodular.

a) 3 and 4 are correct.

b) 2 and 5 are correct.

c) 1 and 3 are correct.

d) 1, 2 and 3 are correct.

e) none of the above are correct.

10. Rectovaginal examination includes palpating

a) the rectovaginal septum.

b) the posterior cul-de-sac.

c) the lateral portions of the pelvis.

d) all of the above.

11. The urethral meatus is examined for

    1. inflammation or lesions.

    2. discharge.

    3. prolapse of the urethral mucosa.

    4. inflammation of Bartholin's glands.

    5. rectocele.

a) 1, 2 and 3 are correct.

b) 2, 3 and 4 are correct.

c) 1, 2 and 4 are correct.

d) 2, 3 and 5 are correct.

e) all of the above are correct.

12. In using the vaginal speculum

    1. commercial lubricants are used when cytological specimens are being obtained.

    2. the blades are inserted obliquely rather than horizontally.

    3. one size is adequate for all women because of the elasticity of the introitus.

    4. it is usually warmed and lubricated with water.

a) 1 and 4 are correct.

b) 2 and 3 are correct.

c) 1 and 2 are correct.

d) 2 and 4 are correct.

e) all of the above are correct.

Match the symptoms in 13 through 17 with the most likely causative factor.

13. _________ Thick, curdy, white vaginal discharge   a) Trichomonas
                                                       b) Monilia
14. _________ Profuse, yellow-green, frothy vaginal discharge   c) Gonorrhea
                                                       d) Senile vaginitis
15. _________ Atrophic, dry, vaginal mucosa

16. _________ Pus draining from the urethra

17. _________ Inflamed vaginal mucosa with white plaques

18. Factors which may cause the client to be apprehensive during the genitourinary and rectal examination include
    1. fear of discovering cancer or venereal disease.
    2. fear of discomfort.
    3. modesty.
    4. not knowing what is going to happen during the examination.
    a) 1, 2 and 4 are correct.
    b) 1 only is correct.
    c) 3 and 4 are correct.
    d) all of the above are correct.

19. The vulva is examined for
    1. color, swelling, lesions of the labia.
    2. distribution of pubic hair.
    3. inflammation of the urethral meatus and vaginal introitus.
    4. strength of perineal muscles.
    5. integrity of hymen.
    a) 1 and 3 are correct.
    b) 1, 3 and 4 are correct.
    c) 2 and 5 are correct.
    d) all of the above are correct.

20. Mrs. Anderson, age 26, is brought to the emergency room in acute distress. Vital signs are BP 90/50, P 120, R 32; skin is cool, clammy and pale. A brief history obtained from her husband states that about 2 hours ago she complained of severe sharp pain in the right lower abdominal quadrant and vomited. Your examination reveals a rigid, tender abdomen. Bimanual palpation demonstrates acute pelvic tenderness but no masses or discharge. Rectal exam is negative. In questioning the husband further, he is unaware of her time in the menstrual cycle, but says that they have been trying to have a baby. The most logical explanation for your client's symptoms is
    a) acute appendicitis.
    b) ruptured tubal pregnancy.
    c) pelvic inflammatory disease.
    d) ovarian cyst.
    e) self-induced abortion.

Number 23

The Genitourinary and Rectal Examination (Female)

RATIONALE

This self-instructional unit is designed to help you learn systematic assessment of the female genitourinary system and rectal area. Primary emphasis is on identifying and describing the normal internal and external structures and recognizing some common abnormalities. Proper use of the vaginal speculum and the procedure for obtaining cytological specimens are stressed.

GLOSSARY OF TERMS

Review the following terms before and after completing this unit. You should be able to define or describe them readily.

Adnexa____

Bartholin's (greater vestibular) glands______________________________

Caruncle____

Chadwick's sign____

Chancre____

Clitoris____

Cystocele____

Dysmenorrhea____

Endometriosis____

Fibroid (myoma)____

Gonorrhea____

Hegar's sign____

Hemorrhoids____

Hymen ____

Leukorrhea ____

Monilia ____

Multipara ____

Nullipara ____

Oophoritis ____

Papanicolaou ____

Perineum ____

Pouch of Douglas ____

Prepuce ____

Rectocele ____

Salpingitis ____

Skene's (paraurethral) glands ________________________________

Trichomonas ____

Vaginitis ____

Vulva ____

COGNITIVE OBJECTIVES

At the end of this unit you will demonstrate knowledge of inspection and palpation of the female genitourinary and rectal areas by your ability to:

1. Name and label the parts of the external and internal female genitalia: mons pubis, labia majora, prepuce, clitoris, labia minora, hymen, vestibule, vaginal introitus, urethral meatus, Bartholin's glands, Skene's glands, perineum, ovaries, fallopian tubes, uterus, cervix, fornix, vagina, rectouterine pouch of Douglas, bladder, urethra, rectum.

2. Discuss preparation of the client for examination and psychosocial aspects associated with assessment of the sexual organs.

3. Describe the normal findings for inspection and palpation of the external genitalia: mons pubis, labia, clitoris, urethral meatus, vestibule, vaginal introitus, hymen.

4. Describe the technique for checking for discharge from Bartholin's and Skene's glands.

5. Give a rationale for and describe the procedure for palpating perineal muscle strength.

6. Discuss selection, preparation and manipulation of the vaginal speculum.

7. Describe normal findings for the vaginal wall, cervix and its os: color, size, placement.

8. List in order and describe the procedures for obtaining cervical cytological specimens: endocervical, ectocervical, vaginal pool.

9. Discuss the purpose and procedure for bimanual examination; describe normal findings for the cervix, fornix, uterus, adnexa: size, shape, consistency, mobility, tenderness of any masses.

10. Describe normal findings for the rectum.

11. Discuss common clinical findings associated with pregnancy and aging.

12. Discuss causative factors, symptoms and clinical signs associated with common abnormal conditions: weakness of the vaginal or pelvic wall, inflammation of glands, trauma, chronic cervicitis, carcinoma, polyps, Trichomonas infection, monilial (Candida) infection, gonorrhea, syphilis, myomas (fibroids), ovarian masses, pelvic inflammatory disease (PID), ruptured tubal pregnancy, endometriosis, hemorrhoids.

LEARNING ACTIVITIES

The Learning Activities contain information necessary for meeting the Cognitive Objectives. Select one and work with it until you have mastered the material. Use the Cognitive Objectives as a study guide. A Self-Test is provided so that you can check how much you know. If you have difficulty with the Self-Test, please review the material in this unit before proceeding to the Clinical Objectives.

Reading Activities

a) Bates: *A Guide to Physical Examination*, "Female Genitalia." This chapter clearly presents written and diagrammed material on basic anatomy of the female genitourinary system, systematic assessment and tables of a few common abnormalities. Findings associated with pregnancy and aging are included. The section on bimanual palpation is especially well done. It is recommended that the student also review the chapter entitled "Anus and Rectum."

b) DeGowin and DeGowin: *Bedside Diagnostic Examination*, pp. 583–604, 498–501. This is the most complete and detailed coverage of genitourinary anatomy, physiology and examination techniques and is recommended for the practitioner seeking in-depth information. Discussion of key signs and symptoms is included throughout the examination procedures.

c) Delp and Manning: *Major's Physical Diagnosis*, "Examination of the Female Genitalia." Knowledge of anatomy and physiology is assumed. The basic examination is well described, and common abnormal findings integrated into the text. The procedure for obtaining Pap smears is not as well explained as in some other readings. This selection is especially helpful in that it covers the patient history and includes a glossary.

d) Gillies and Alyn: *Patient Assessment and Management by the Nurse Practitioner*, pp. 100–101, 103–107. Knowledge of anatomical location of external and internal structures is assumed. This reading provides an overview of examination procedures and findings. Supplementation is needed in all areas to meet the objectives.

e) Judge and Zuidema: *Methods of Clinical Examination: A Physiologic Approach*, "The Female Reproductive System." Knowledge of anatomy is assumed. This chapter presents a very readable overview of procedures and normal findings. The climate for the examination and client approach are well covered. Supplement your learning in all other areas.

f) Prior and Silberstein: *Physical Diagnosis*, "Genitalia," pp. 312–330. A comprehensive discussion of examination procedures with emphasis on normal findings. If collection of cytological specimens is a new procedure to you, supplement your learning with a more detailed explanation of the techniques involved.

g) Sana and Judge: *Physical Appraisal Methods in Nursing Practice*, Chapter 12, "Physical Appraisal of the Female Reproductive System." Familiarity with anatomy is assumed. Assessment of the external and internal genitalia is brief and concise. Information on findings of the postmenopausal woman is included. Supplement your learning to include pertinent anatomy, common abnormalities and rectal findings.

h) Sherman and Fields: *Guide to Patient Evaluation*. This selection covers pertinent anatomy and physiology, examination techniques and normal findings. An example of charting for this examination is included and may be helpful. Additional reading is suggested to supply more in-depth information about abnormalities.

Audiovisual Activities

a) Blue-Hill Educational Systems, Inc.: "The Gynecologic Examination – Part XIV," a video tape cassette. This comprehensive presentation in lecture format covers anatomy and physiology, systematic examination, obtaining cytological specimens and bimanual palpation. Normal and abnormal findings are included. The student will also need to view the last part of the film, "The Abdomen – Part XIII," for information on the rectal examination.

b) Ortho Pharmaceutical Co. OMNI series: "Pelvic Examination." This self-instructional learning activity combines reading, 35-mm slides, films and simulated practice to present a complete coverage of the pelvic examination for use by nurses who are learning expanded roles in OB-GYN educational programs.

Supplemental Activity

The following material is suggested to strengthen your learning.

a) Eli Lilly Co.: "Female Pelvic Examination." This color film demonstrates examination of external genitalia, use of speculum, Pap smears, bimanual palpation. Abnormal findings are included.

SELF-TEST

This Self-Test is for you. Use it to check how well you have learned the material presented in this unit. The answers follow the test.

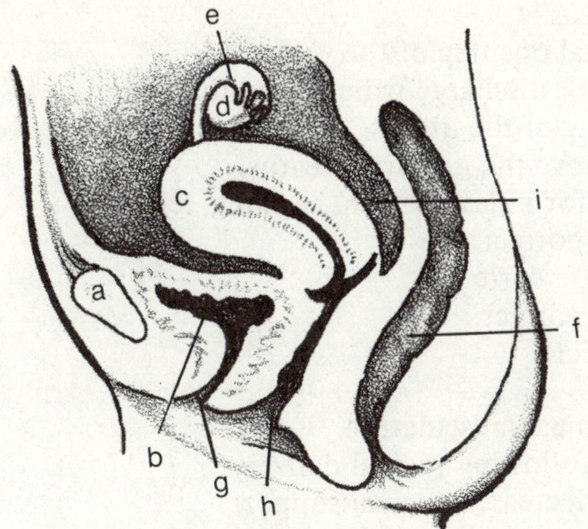

1. Identify the structures indicated on the accompanying diagram.

a) _______________________________   f) _______________________________

b) _______________________________   g) _______________________________

c) _______________________________   h) _______________________________

d) _______________________________   i) _______________________________

e) _______________________________

2. To help your client relax during the examination you should
    1. have her empty her bladder.
    2. provide a small head pillow.
    3. provide privacy and drape adequately.
    4. explain purpose and steps in the examination after performing them.
    a) 3 only is correct.
    b) 1, 2 and 3 are correct.
    c) 2 and 4 are correct.
    d) all of the above are correct.

3. The term commonly used to refer to the external genitalia is
    a) vestibule.
    b) mons pubis.
    c) perineum.
    d) vulva.
    e) adnexa.

4. The external genitalia are examined for
    1. distribution of pubic hair.
    2. size, contour and color.
    3. swelling, lesions.
    4. discharge from urethra, vagina and glands.

    a)   2 and 3 are correct.
    b)   1 and 4 are correct.
    c)   1, 3 and 4 are correct.
    d)   all of the above are correct.

5. The vaginal introitus is
      1.   the external opening of the vagina.
      2.   palpated for discharge from Bartholin's glands.
      3.   the opening of the uterus.
      4.   located above the urethral meatus.
      5.   inspected for inflammation, swelling, lesions.
    a)   1, 4 and 5 are correct.
    b)   2, 3, 4 and 5 are correct.
    c)   1, 2 and 5 are correct.
    d)   3 only is correct.

6. Relaxation of perineal musculature
      1.   is normal following vaginal delivery.
      2.   results in decreased vaginal support.
      3.   if extensive may allow bulging of the bladder into the vagina.
      4.   if extensive can lead to rectocele.
    a)   1 only is correct.
    b)   1, 2 and 3 are correct.
    c)   2 and 4 are correct.
    d)   all of the above are correct.

7. The vaginal speculum is usually
      1.   warmed and lubricated with water.
      2.   inserted horizontally.
      3.   inserted with the blades held partly open by the thumb lever.
      4.   withdrawn from the vagina with the blades completely closed.
      5.   held open by tightening the thumb screw during examination.
    a)   1 and 5 are correct.
    b)   1, 3, 4 and 5 are correct.
    c)   2, 3, 4 and 5 are correct.
    d)   1, 2, 4 and 5 are correct.
    e)   1 only is correct.

8. The recommended order in which cervical cytological specimens are obtained is
    a)   vaginal pool, endocervical, ectocervical.
    b)   ectocervical, vaginal pool, endocervical.
    c)   endocervical, ectocervical, vaginal pool.
    d)   ectocervical, endocervical, vaginal pool.

9. Bimanual palpation is performed to assess
    a)   the size, shape, consistency and mobility of the uterus.
    b)   characteristics of the adnexal areas.
    c)   both a and b.

10. Thick, white, curdy vaginal discharge and an inflamed vaginal mucosa with white
     plaques is characteristic of
    a)   Trichomonas infection
    b)   syphilis

    c) gonorrhea.
    d) carcinoma.
    e) monilial infection

11. Rectal examination is an important part of the examination for
    a) detecting cancer of the rectum.
    b) palpating the posterior aspect of the uterus.
    c) assessing rectal sphincter tone.
    d) evaluating the stool for occult blood.
    e) all of the above.

SELF-TEST KEY

1. (a) symphysis pubis   (f) rectum
    (b) bladder   (g) urethra
    (c) uterus   (h) vagina
    (d) ovary   (i) pouch of Douglas
    (e) fallopian tube

2. (b) A full bladder not only will make the examination uncomfortable for your client but also may be mistaken for a pregnant uterus or mass. Draping and screening from the doorway are important considerations in promoting relaxation. Avoid any interruptions during the examination. A small pillow under the head helps to relax the abdominal muscles. The purpose of the examination and steps in the procedures should be explained prior to performing them so that your client will know what to expect. This also provides a good opportunity to assess needs for teaching or reassurance.

3. (d) The external genitalia (mons pubis, labia, prepuce, clitoris and vestibule) are collectively referred to as the vulva. The perineum refers to the tissue between the anus and vaginal introitus. The adnexa are composed of the uterine appendages: ovaries, tubes and supporting ligaments.

4. (d) The external genitalia are inspected for normal distribution of sexual hair and development of structures. Swellings or lesions are palpated to determine induration. and tenderness. The glands are palpated to check for inflammation and discharge. If infection is suspected, the urethra is "milked" to obtain discharge for culture.

5. (c) The vaginal introitus is the opening of the vagina which leads up to the cervix and uterus. It is observed for inflammation, swelling, lesions and discharge. Palpation of the introitus between thumb and forefinger allows assessment of Bartholin's glands for inflammation and discharge. The introitus is located below the urethral meatus.

6. (d) Following vaginal delivery, there is decreased tone of the perineal muscles due to stretching. Normally this resolves without incidence. If there is extensive damage or the muscles are continually stretched with numerous pregnancies, the pelvic organs will bulge into the vagina. Weakness of the anterior wall allows the bladder to bulge into the vagina (cystocele); posterior weakness leads to rectocele from pressure of the rectum against the wall.

7. (a) The speculum is warmed and lubricated with water. The closed blades are inserted obliquely and then rotated into a horizontal position. Pressure on the thumb

lever opens the blades which are then fixed in position by the thumb screw. For withdrawal, the thumb screw is released, and separation of the blades is maintained by thumb pressure so that the vaginal walls can be inspected. Premature closure of the blades will pinch the cervix.

8. (c) A saline-moistened cotton swab is rotated in the cervical os to obtain the endocervical specimen; next, a vaginal spatula with long end in the os scrapes the cervix; finally, a spatula or cotton swab is used to sample the "pool" beneath the cervix.

9. (c) Bimanual palpation allows the examiner to gain additional information about the uterus and its appendages (ovaries, tubes, supporting ligaments) in the adnexal areas.

10. (e) Characteristics of monilial infection (*Candida albicans*) include a thick, white, curdy discharge and reddened mucosa with white or gray patches; frequently, the client complains of itching or burning vulva.

11. (e) The rectal examination is a simple method for early detection of rectal carcinoma. Rectovaginal bimanual palpation supplies additional information about the uterus and adnexal areas. Additionally, the examiner is able to check for laxity or abnormal tightness of the rectal sphincter. Stool which adheres to the gloves is easily checked for occult blood.

CLINICAL COMPONENT

Having completed the cognitive portion of this unit, you are now ready to proceed to the Clinical Objectives. The purpose of the Clinical Component is to help you learn to assess the female genitourinary structures and rectum for normal configuration and function, obtain cytological specimens and detect the presence, location and extent of any dysfunction.

CLINICAL OBJECTIVES

At the end of this unit you will perform genitourinary and rectal assessment, correlating physical examination skills with physiological principles. You will be able to:

1. Demonstrate knowledge of signs and symptoms of dysfunction related to the genitourinary and rectal systems by obtaining a pertinent health history from the client.

2. Demonstrate an understanding of the psychosocial implications of examination of the sexual organs by properly preparing the client.

3. Demonstrate inspection of the external genitalia by systematically assessing the vulva.

4. Demonstrate palpation of Bartholin's glands.

5. Test perineal muscle strength.

6. Demonstrate proper selection, preparation and manipulation of the speculum.

7. Systematically assess the cervix and its os as to color and position.

8. Correctly obtain and prepare three specimens for cytological examination.

9. Assess the characteristics of the vaginal wall.

10. Perform bimanual examination – vaginal and rectovaginal.

11. Utilize the S.O.A.P. method of recording to systematically describe findings, make an assessment regarding normality and formulate a plan of action.

INSTRUCTIONS

Practice with the vaginal speculum until you can open, close and adjust the blades easily.
Utilizing three of your peers or clients in the clinical area, practice inspection and palpation of the vulva, manipulation of the speculum to inspect the vagina and cervix and obtain cytological specimens and bimanual palpation of the internal pelvic organs. Remove Performance Guide cards for Unit 23 from Appendix II. These cards will enable you to practice the skills necessary to meet the Clinical Objectives and complete the Response Sheets. You will be expected to (1) ask questions which may elicit possible symptoms, (2) systematically describe your findings, (3) localize any abnormalities present and (4) summarize your examination findings using the S.O.A.P. method of recording.
When you have mastered the Clinical Objectives and completed the Response Sheets, arrange to demonstrate your skills to your laboratory instructor or preceptor.

EQUIPMENT

Cotton-tipped swabs, vaginal spatulas, glass slides and fixative for specimens
Disposable gloves
Drape
Examination table with stirrups
Movable light
Small pillow
Tissues (for post-exam cleansing)
Vaginal speculum (several sizes)

OPTIONAL ACTIVITIES

These activities demonstrate techniques for assessment of the female genitourinary and rectal system.
a) Bates: "Female Genitalia, Anus and Rectum" (film).
b) Eli Lilly Co.: "Female Pelvic Examination." This color film (approximately 20 minutes) presents a clear and concise live demonstration of examination of the external genitalia, use of the speculum for inspecting the cervix and obtaining Pap smears and bimanual palpation. Abnormal findings are included.
c) OMNI (Ortho Pharmaceutical Corp.): Simulated pelvic model, "Gynny."
d) Blue-Hill Educational Systems, Inc.: "Gynecologic," a video tape cassette which is approximately 16 minutes long.

RESPONSE SHEET—GENITOURINARY AND RECTAL EXAMINATION (FEMALE)

Client _______________________________________

Date ________________ Age ___________________

Examiner _____________________________________

I. Health History

II. Physical Examination

   A. External Genitalia

      1. Vulva

         a. Mons pubis

         b. Labia majora

         c. Perineum

      2. Vestibule

         a. Labia minora

         b. Clitoris

         c. Urethral meatus

         d. Vaginal introitus

3. Perineal muscle strength

B. Internal Genitalia

1. Cervix

2. Pap smears: endocervical________, cervical scrape________, vaginal pool________

3. Vaginal mucosa

C. Bimanual Examination

1. Vaginal wall

2. Cervix

3. Uterus

4. Adnexa

D. Rectal Examination

Summarize your findings using the S.O.A.P. method.

S. (Client's observations, complaints, health history)

O. (Physical findings)

A. (Assessment of the problem, data, prognosis)

P. (Plans for further evaluation, care, teaching)

Client _______________________________

Date _________________ Age _______________

Examiner _______________________________

I. Health History

II. Physical Examination

A. External Genitalia

1. Vulva

   a. Mons pubis

   b. Labia majora

   c. Perineum

2. Vestibule

   a. Labia minora

   b. Clitoris

   c. Urethral meatus

   d. Vaginal introitus

    3. Perineal muscle strength

B. Internal Genitalia

    1. Cervix

    2. Pap smears: endocervical _______, cervical scrape _______, vaginal pool _______

    3. Vaginal mucosa

C. Bimanual Examination

    1. Vaginal wall

    2. Cervix

    3. Uterus

    4. Adnexa

D. Rectal Examination

Summarize your findings using the S.O.A.P. method.

S. (Client's observations, complaints, health history)

O. (Physical findings)

A. (Assessment of the problem, data, prognosis)

P. (Plans for further evaluation, care, teaching)

RESPONSE SHEET—GENITOURINARY AND RECTAL EXAMINATION (FEMALE)

Client _______________________________

Date _________________ Age _____________

Examiner _____________________________

I. Health History

II. Physical Examination

   A. External Genitalia

      1. Vulva

         a. Mons pubis

         b. Labia majora

         c. Perineum

      2. Vestibule

         a. Labia minora

         b. Clitoris

         c. Urethral meatus

         d. Vaginal introitus

3. Perineal muscle strength

B. Internal Genitalia

1. Cervix

2. Pap smears: endocervical________, cervical scrape________, vaginal pool________

3. Vaginal mucosa

C. Bimanual Examination

1. Vaginal wall

2. Cervix

3. Uterus

4. Adnexa

D. Rectal Examination

Summarize your findings using the S.O.A.P. method.

S. (Client's observations, complaints, health history)

O. (Physical findings)

A. (Assessment of the problem, data, prognosis)

P. (Plans for further evaluation, care, teaching)

EXAMPLES OF
PROBLEM-ORIENTED CHARTING

CLIENT PROBLEM LIST

Jones, Martha

01-02-003

Examiner: S.L. Rush, R.N.

Date Recorded	Active	Inactive
3/7/76 #1	Acute pelvic inflammatory disease	
#2	Allergy to pollen, feathers, animal fur	
#3	Unfamiliar with breast self-exam	
#4		Appendectomy – 1970
#5		Abortion – 1975
#6		Depression (situational) – 1975

INITIAL PLANS

Patient   Jones, Martha

Date   01-02-003

Examiner S.L. Rush, R.N.

Problem #1	Acute pelvic inflammatory disease
Diagnostic plan	Per algorithm: Established by history, pelvic and rectal examination and positive gram-negative stain of cervical and urethral secretions. Smears of cervical, urethral and anal secretions to lab for culture and sensitivity. Epidemiology slip routed to Public Health.
Therapeutic plan	Per protocol: Procaine penicillin G, 4.8 million units IM. Probenecid, 1 gm, po, ½ hr after penicillin. Doxycycline (Vibramycin), 100 mg bid X 10 days. Bedrest at home. Return tomorrow if not improved. Return in 1 week for re-evaluation.
Client education	Explained that pain was due to inflammation of fallopian tubes. Advised against intercourse or douching during treatment. Reaffirmed her suspicion of probable gonococcal infection. Advised to inform sex partner of possible diagnosis and encourage him to seek treatment. Informed that epidemiological report will be sent to health dept. and that she will be contacted by an investigator. First dose of doxycycline at bedtime or when nausea and vomiting subside. Informed not to take med with milk or snacks, as food tends to inhibit absorption of medication.

PROGRESS NOTES

Patient Problem*

Patient: Mrs. T. F., age 65.
Chief complaint: "Very short of breath."
Problem: Cardiac murmur and left-sided heart failure.

S. Good general health. No history of rheumatic fever. Systolic murmur noted at age 38 but no symptoms until 1 yr ago. Progressively worse SOB with two episodes of PND within past week. No ankle edema.

O. BP 180/80 Pulse 100, vigorous beat. Pulses visible.
Inspection – Carotid pulse visible and pulsation noted in suprasternal notch. Apical impulse in 6th LICS, 3 cm lateral to MCL with retraction of interspaces, not ribs.
Palpation – PMI forceful at location of apical impulses, slight lift at apex. Diastolic thrill between left sternal border and MCL in 3rd and 4th LICS. Liver not enlarged.
Percussion – No pulmonary dullness. LBCD maximal in 6th LICS, 4 cm lateral to MCL.
Auscultation – Bilateral basal rales, posteriorly. A_2 accentuated. $A_2 > P_2$. Other sounds normal. Blowing, high-pitched decrescendo grade 4/6 murmur, beginning just after A_2 and disappearing in late diastole, heard best at Erb's point, radiating up to aortic area, carotid vessels, downward to apex. No gallop.

A. Probable aortic insufficiency with early left-sided heart failure.

P. Refer to cardiologist promptly.

---

*From Sherman, J.L., and Fields, S.K.: *A Guide to Patient Evaluation*. Flushing, N.Y., Medical Examination Publishing Company, Inc., 1974, pp. 150–151.

PROGRESS NOTES

Patient Problem*

Ms. S.D., a 22-yr-old, well-developed, white, married grav. 0, para 0 female, with "vaginal itch, burning on urination and vaginal discharge," of 1 week's duration.

Problem: Pruritus, dysuria, vaginal discharge.

S. Treated with erythromycin 4 weeks ago for RUL pneumonia. Was well until 7 days ago when she first noticed increased vaginal discharge with severe itch and burning on urination. Has taken Ovulen for birth control past 2 yr, no untoward effects. Menses of 28 days ± 3 days, no dysmenorrhea, no clots or spotting, uses 4 tampons qd. No dyspareunia. Urine neg. for sugar in hospital. No family history of diabetes.

O. Vestibule and urethra red and irritated.
Vagina – Reddened mucosa, white curds clinging to wall.
Uterus, cervix and adnexa with normal limits
Discharge – Thin, watery 2+, no odor.
Pap – Done (to lab).
Urine – Neg. sugar.
Wet prep – No trichomonads seen, cells typical of *Monilia albicans.*

A. In view of recent Rx with erythromycin, increased susceptibility due to Ovulen, typical monilia cells seen on wet prep, suggest *Monilia albicans* vaginitis.

P. Dx – 2 hr pc blood sugar.
Rx – Mycostatin suppositories bid X 4 days and then hs 1 week.
Pt. Ed. – Advise to avoid sexual intercourse, use of tampons, and douching for 2 weeks. If not cleared, return for consultation.

---

*From Sherman, J.L., and Fields, S.K.: *A Guide to Patient Evaluation.* Flushing, N.Y., Medical Examination Publishing Company, Inc., 1974, pp. 202–203.

Appendix II

PERFORMANCE GUIDES

These Performance Guides will enable you to practice the skills necessary to meet the clinical objectives for each unit or group of units. The guides may also be used as organizational aids during examinations. They are designed so that you can detach the appropriate page(s) for the corresponding instructional units and cut them into individual cards for convenient use.

UNIT 2—THE HEALTH HISTORY

GENERAL INSTRUCTIONS

1. Conduct interview in pleasant nonthreatening environment, preferably a quiet, private room.
2. Conduct interview shortly after client's arrival.
3. Open interview with courteous greeting; give name, title, status.
4. Begin by eliciting reasons client is seeking health care. "Tell me, how might I help you?"
5. Initially utilize open-ended questions to allow client to express thoughts and feelings.
6. Observe for nonverbal communication.
7. Use vocabulary the client understands.
8. Listen carefully, without bias or judgment; concentrate on facts and feelings.
9. Maintain interested, supportive attitude.
10. Use direct questioning to clarify data in specific area.

CHIEF COMPLAINT

1. Determine client's major concern and its duration.
2. Record complaint briefly (in client's words) — e.g., "black stools," 7 days' duration.
3. Do not translate client concern into a diagnosis.

PRESENT ILLNESS

1. Determine onset, chronology of events, current status and reasons for seeking health care now. "Tell me as much as you remember from the time this problem began until now."
2. Seek description of symptoms.
   Type — Shortness of breath, nausea, fatigue, pain (stabbing, burning, throbbing).
   Severity — How do symptoms affect daily activity?
   Duration — Length of single attack and frequency of symptom over period of time.

Continued

PRESENT ILLNESS—*Continued*

Influencing factors — Can client identify factors which precipitate symptom (e.g., walking upstairs)? What actions relieve symptom (resting in bed)? Does it occur generally at the same time of day or season of year? Is it associated with position (standing, sitting, stretching)? Is it associated with other events (eating, emotional upsets, alcohol intake, coughing)?

3. Record systematically, using narrative format.

PAST MEDICAL HISTORY

1. Redirect interview toward other medical or surgical problems. "How would you describe your health before this problem began?" "Tell me about other illnesses or operations you have had."
2. Direct questioning may be needed in some areas to clarify client perceptions or elicit information client sees as insignificant or anxiety-provoking.
3. Record entries with dates of occurrence, severity and complications, if any. Record only established diagnoses.
4. Record current medications, immunizations, allergies. A drug allergy is an important active problem on every problem list.

FAMILY HISTORY

1. Question client about age and current health status of parents, siblings, children.
2. Question client about age at death and cause of death of parents, siblings, children.
3. Inquire about exposure to tuberculosis. Utilize history form to ascertain occurrence of specific disease entities among family members.

PERSONAL AND SOCIAL HISTORY

1. Shift interview back to client. You can do this by asking client "Where were you born?" "Are you married?" "What is your present occupation?"
2. Concentrate on facts and feelings expressed by the client.
3. Request information about client's habits, diet, occupation, education, daily stresses, hobbies.
4. Solicit information about client's daily routine.
5. Utilize this information to evaluate client holistically.

UNIT 3–EXAMINATION OF THE INTEGUMENT

3A

GENERAL INFORMATION

1. Diffuse overhead fluorescent lighting is best.
2. Client should be properly draped to preserve modesty.
3. With client sitting on exam table, observe exposed areas and back; with client supine, systematically move drape to inspect other areas.
4. Examination of mucous membranes recorded with EENT exam.
5. *All* lesions are examined with *gloves*. Culture any suspicious lesions. Note character of exudates.

HEALTH HISTORY: Ask client about

1. Past Hx of dermatological problems — onset, recurrence, site(s), characteristics of lesions, associated Sx's, Rx (self, drugs, surgery, cosmetics).
2. Current problems — lesions (characteristics), pain, pruritus (localized, generalized), photosensitivity, allergies, current medications (vitamins, hormones), other medical problems, trauma.
3. Habits — hygiene, diet, sleep, cosmetics, exposure to irritants (geographical, occupational, household).

SKIN

3B

1. Color — pigment, cyanosis, pallor, jaundice, flush.
2. Vascularity — evidence of bruising, bleeding; vascular and purpuric lesions (angioma, petechia, purpura).
3. Lesions
Type — Primary: macule, papule, plaque, nodule, tumor, wheal, vesicle, bulla, pustule. *Secondary:* erosion, ulcer, fissure, crust, scale, lichenification, atrophy, excoriation, scars.
Grouping — clustered, linear, annular.
Distribution — localized, generalized, exposed.
4. Moisture — dryness, sweating, oiliness.
5. Temperature (use back of your hand to test).
6. Texture — rough, smooth.
7. Mobility and turgor — lift fold of skin, see how easily it falls back into place; thickness, edema.

SYSTEMS REVIEW

2E

1. Utilize health history form to review all past and current symptoms experienced by client.
2. This review provides a check on the completeness of information in present and past histories.
3. Question client directly, using words client understands.
4. Negative responses are recorded as such. Positive responses require explanations and details.

NAILS

3C

1. Color, shape, angle between nail and base (clubbing).
2. Ridges, lesions (splinter hemorrhages).

HAIR

1. Texture, luster, quantity, distribution.
2. Examine scalp for dandruff, lesions.

UNIT 4–EXAMINATION OF THE PERIPHERAL VASCULAR SYSTEM 4A

GENERAL INSTRUCTIONS

1. Observe client's color, respirations and emotional state for clues before beginning exam.
2. If client is anxious or BP elevated, repeat measurements in 15 min.
3. Use correct size BP cuff; average adult, 12–14 cm wide; obese arm or thigh, 18–20 cm; child or thin arm, less than 12 cm or pediatric size.
4. Do not take measurement over clothing.
5. Sphygmomanometer should be at heart level.
6. 5–10 mm Hg difference between arms is normal. Systolic pressure normally higher in thighs than arms.
7. If unable to auscultate BP, have client elevate arm over head for few minutes (decreases venous pressure).
8. For examination of pulses use tangential lighting.

BLOOD PRESSURE 4C

Compare measurements in both arms with client standing, sitting, supine.

1. Palpation — Wrap cuff over upper arm. Palpate brachial artery, inflate cuff 20 mm Hg higher than you can feel the pulse.
2. Auscultation — Use diaphragm; palpate brachial artery for systolic and then auscultate, release cuff 3–5 mm Hg at a time. Use Korotkoff method to record BP:

Onset of sound (systole).
Auscultatory gap (no sound).
Distinct sounds.
Muffled sounds.
Disappearance of sound. } Record both for diastole (e.g., 120/80/76).
Thigh pressure — Amputees, burns.
Large cuff over distal 1/3; client prone with leg slightly elevated; auscultate popliteal artery.

HEALTH HISTORY: Ask client about 4B

1. Weight gain, shortness of breath, orthopnea, fatigue, chest pain, palpitations, wheezing, high BP, tingling, fainting, leg cramps, edema, claudication, varicose veins, cold or blue feet, nitroglycerin, digitalis, diuretics, BP medications.

NECK VESSELS 4D

1. Carotid artery — Medial border of sternocleidomastoid muscle.
Inspection — Look for monophasic pressure wave simultaneous with apical heart beat (PMI). Compare for symmetry.
Palpation — Hook fingers around sternocleidomastoid muscle, avoid pressure on carotid sinus (at level of thyroid cartilage), palpate only *one* side at a time. Note rate, rhythm, amplitude, contour; symmetry.
2. Internal jugular vein — Diffuse triphasic pressure wave (a, c, v waves). Transmitted to surrounding tissue.
Inspection — Observe for pulse at suprasternal notch with client supine and head slightly elevated. If jugular veins appear distended, observe for changes associated with respiration (normally flatten with inspiration) and with gradual elevation of the head to 45° (normally do not fill above clavicles at 45°). Estimate venous pressure by measuring vertical distance between fluid level and sternal angle.
Palpation — Pulse easily occluded by light pressure.

Continued

NECK VESSELS—*Continued* 4E

If vessels distended, perform following tests:

Direction of blood flow — Place one thumb above the other over jugular, strip vessel in both directions to flatten, release one thumb and observe direction of flow (normally from head to heart).

HJR — Tell patient to keep breathing at normal rate and depth; apply firm pressure with one hand on top of other over right upper quadrant of abdomen, pushing down and superiorly for 30 seconds; observe elevation in height of fluid column in vein.

PERIPHERAL VESSELS

1. Arteries

Inspection — Note any visible pulsations.

Palpation — Check for rate, rhythm or regularity, amplitude or force (absent, weak, normal, strong, bounding), symmetry. Proceed from body to periphery: *brachial, radial, femoral* (deep, ½ way between anterior sup. iliac

Continued

PERIPHERAL VESSELS—*Continued* 4F

crest and pubic tubercle), *popliteal* (client prone, flex knee slightly; feel deep, lateral to midline in popliteal fossa), *posterior tibial* (stand in front, feel behind and below medial maleolus of ankle), *dorsalis pedis* (top of foot, medial to tendon over arch).

Be alert to signs of arterial insufficiency: decreased or absent pulses; thin, shiny, atrophic skin, loss of hair, discoloration, ulcerations, gangrene, long venous filling time (occlude artery with thumb pressure until blanches, release pressure, note time for skin to become pink again), cool extremity.

2. Veins

Inspection — Superficial varicosities (usually on legs), swelling, redness.

Palpation — Check for pitting if edema noted. Check for signs of deep thrombosis: swelling (measure both legs), temperature, cords, pain (press calf against leg bones), Homans' sign (slightly flex knee, dorsiflex foot manually; pain = positive result). Note: a shortened Achilles tendon will also produce discomfort.

UNIT 5–MUSCULOSKELETAL EXAMINATION 5A

GENERAL INSTRUCTIONS

1. Client wears minimal clothing to facilitate examiner's view of muscle/joint motion. Be sure room temperature is comfortable.

2. Work in systematic order: general appearance, head and neck, extremities, spine. Compare symmetrical points. Measure difference in muscle or joint size or limb length with tape measure.

3. Abnormal findings dictate a more extensive exam. If trauma suspected, postpone exam until x-rays are read. Be especially careful of spinal injuries.

HEALTH HISTORY: Ask client about

1. History of trauma, surgery, arthritis, gout; medications.

2. Amount of physical activity, lifting heavy objects, sports (baseball, tennis, skiing), wearing high heels or clogs; back brace, knee support.

3. Current problems: *Joints* — pain, heat, redness, stiffness, deformity. *Muscles* — myalgias, cramps, weakness. Limitation of normal daily activities. Difficulty with or abnormal gait, balance.

GENERAL FUNCTION, POSTURE AND GAIT 5B

1. Throughout examination observe client's ability to perform normal functions: to sit down, stand up, lie down, climb onto exam table, undress, fasten buttons.

2. Gait — Have barefoot client walk away from and toward you. Watch foot placement, width of stance, size and speed of steps, arm swing, position of torso, ability to start and stop easily, need to watch feet placement, need for support, abnormal position or movements of extremities.

3. Use of cane, walker; prosthesis; corrective shoes.

HEAD AND NECK (Client seated)

1. Inspection — Deformities, abnormal posture.

2. Palpation — Swelling, tenderness, crepitation, range.

Temporomandibular joint — Swelling, tenderness. Have client open and close mouth; feel and listen for crepitations, observe ROM.

Tenderness of cervical spine, paravertebral and trapezius muscles?

ROM — Have client touch chin to chest, each shoulder; touch ear to shoulder; extend head backward.

| **HANDS AND WRISTS** 5C | **KNEES** (Legs extended, relaxed) 5E |

HANDS AND WRISTS 5C

1. Inspection — missing, deformed fingers; contractures, swelling, redness, bony enlargements, nodules, atrophy.
2. Palpate all bones in wrist, hand and fingers for tenderness, nodules.
3. ROM — Have client open and close fist; flex, extend, abduct and adduct wrist. Note range, pain, crepitations.

ELBOWS

1. Inspection — deformities, nodules, swelling, redness.
2. Palpation — flex elbow at 70° angle, palpate the groove on either side of the olecranon for swelling, fluid, nodules, tenderness.
3. ROM — Flex and extend forearm, supinate and pronate palms; note range, pain, crepitations.

KNEES (Legs extended, relaxed) 5E

1. Inspection — Inflammation, swelling, enlargement (absence of normal concavities on each side of patella); alignment, deformity.
2. Palpate suprapatellar pouch and downward on either side of patella; note bogginess, thickening, tenderness.
3. ROM — Extension/flexion; note range, pain, crepitations.

HIPS (Client lying flat)

1. Inspection — Is one leg longer than other or abnormally rotated?
2. Palpate along joint for tenderness.
3. ROM — Flex knee firmly onto chest (flexion of opposite thigh indicates deformity of that hip). Touch foot to opposite patella and pull knee laterally and medially to check hip rotation; note range, tenderness, crepitations.

SHOULDERS 5D

1. Inspection — swelling, deformity, atrophy.
2. Palpate sternoclavicular joint at sternum, acromioclavicular joint between clavicle and shoulder, and grooves and head of humerus for tenderness, nodules, fluid.
3. ROM — Have client raise arms over head, put hands behind small of back; note range, crepitations, pain.

FEET AND ANKLES

1. Inspect ankles, foot bones, toes; note deformities, nodules, redness, swelling, fleshy or bony growths.
2. Palpate for tenderness, nodules.
3. ROM — Dorsiflexion and plantar flexion of foot; flex toes, evert and invert foot while holding ankle still, evert and invert forefoot while holding heel still. Note range, tenderness, crepitations.

SPINE (Client standing) 5F

1. Inspection — observe from side to note cervical, thoracic, lumbar curvature; stand behind and look for abnormal lateral curvature, check height of shoulders and iliac crests; does client have flat feet; knock-knees or bowlegs?
2. Palpate firmly along spinous processes for tenderness or muscle spasm.
3. ROM (from behind, stabilize client's hips with your hands) — Have client bend forward and touch toes, bend to each side, twist shoulders from side to side; bend backward. Deformities of spine frequently become more obvious during these maneuvers. Also note range, pain.

UNIT 6–NEUROLOGICAL EXAMINATION   6A

HEALTH HISTORY

1. History of medical Rx, surgery, injuries, allergies, medications, immunizations, hypertension.

2. Current problems — Syncope, seizures, dizziness, memory loss, nervousness, depression, headache, stiff neck, disturbances of hearing, vision, swallowing, weakness, tumors, hyper- or hypoesthesia.

GENERAL CEREBRAL FUNCTIONS   6B

1. *General behavior* — Defects in learned/cultural aspects of behavior? Eccentricities, cooperation.

2. *Levels of consciousness* — Alert → comatose.

3. *Intellectual performance*
Test memory for past events.
Test present memory by asking client to repeat a series of numbers forward and backward.
Check orientation: person, place, time.
Abstract reasoning: have client explain familiar slogan.

4. *Emotional status* — Tension; depression or euphoria.

5. *Thought content* — Preoccupations, inappropriate or obsessive thoughts or ideas.

6. *Cerebral integration* — evaluate ability to
Recognize objects by sight, hearing, touch.
Carry out purposeful, skilled motor movements.
Understand and communicate speech and writing.

CRANIAL NERVES   6C

Olfactory nerve (I)
Test with client's eyes closed. Have client identify familiar odors such as coffee, cloves.
Optic nerve (II)

1. Test visual acuity with Snellen chart or newspaper.

2. Test visual fields: Client covers one eye and looks at the examiner. (Examiner covers own opposite eye and compares field of vision with client's.) Starting at periphery of each quadrant of vision, examiner moves finger toward client's center of vision. Client indicates when he sees finger. Repeat for other side.

Oculomotor (III), *trochlear* (IV), *and abducens* (VI) *nerves* (Oculomotor nerve also constricts pupils and elevates lids.)

1. Ocular movements — Client follows examiner's finger as it is moved in all directions.

Abnormal III — Unable to look up, down, or horizontally nasal; ptosis, dilation of pupil.

Continued

CRANIAL NERVES—*Continued*   6D

Abnormal IV — Unable to look nasally downward.
Abnormal VI — Unable to look horizontally temporal.

2. Check for nystagmus, lid lag, ptosis.

3. Pupillary accommodation reflex — Check constriction as client changes focus from distant to close object. Pupils should also converge equally.

4. Check direct and consensual constriction to light.

Trigeminal nerve (V) — Note any asymmetry.

1. Touch forehead, cheeks and jaw with wisp of cotton. Failure to feel indicates anesthesia.

2. Repeat procedure in 1, checking for temperature sense.

3. Lightly touch cornea with wisp of cotton (corneal reflex) to initiate blinking response.

4. Test ability to open jaw against resistance.

Continued

CRANIAL NERVES—*Continued*   6E

Facial nerve (VII)
1. Note ability to wrinkle forehead, frown, smile, raise eyebrows. Note any asymmetry.
2. Identify sugar and/or salt on anterior aspect of tongue on each side (tongue protruded).
Acoustic nerve (VIII)
1. Hearing — Indicate distance client can hear watch tick or speech.
2. Weber test — Place tuning fork on midline of skull. Sound should not lateralize.
3. Rinne test — Place base of tuning fork on mastoid process (bone conduction) until client can no longer hear sound. Then hold fork next to ear to check air conduction (normal: air conduction greater than bone conduction).
4. Abnormal: Tinnitus, decreased hearing or deafness.

Continued

CEREBELLAR FUNCTION: Assess client's ability to   6G

1. Touch finger to nose (eyes open), alternating hands. (Repeat with eyes closed.)
2. Touch finger to nose and then to examiner's moving finger.
3. Run each heel down opposite shin (lying or standing).
4. Rapidly pat knees, alternating back of hands and palms.
5. Stand erect with feet together, first with eyes open, then eyes closed (Romberg test).
In each test observe for actions carried out accurately and smoothly without tremor or ataxia. Note erectness of posture, balance, ability to gauge distance, arm swing.

CRANIAL NERVES—*Continued*   6F

Glossopharyngeal (IX) *and vagus* (X) *nerves*
1. Check for symmetrical rise of uvula with phonation. Abnormal, deviates to unaffected side.
2. Gag reflex — Touch side of pharynx.
3. Normal function of vagus nerve alone is revealed by ability to swallow and to speak clearly.
Accessory nerve (XI)
Palpate strength of trapezius muscle by having client shrug shoulders against resistance.
Hypoglossal nerve (XII)
Note any lateral deviation of protruded tongue; test strength against tongue depressor. Note atrophy or tremor.

MOTOR SYSTEM   6H

1. Mass — Measure arms, thighs, calves; look for wasting, fasciculations, fine tremors.
2. Tone — Note resistance to passive range of motion; look for spasticity, rigidity, flaccidity.
3. Involuntary movements — Tremor at rest, tics, twitching? Examiner extends and flexes client's ankle or elbow; continued repetitive movement when examiner stops indicates clonus.
4. Strength — Test flexion, extension and other movements through major joints, first without resistance and then with examiner offering resistance. Compare each side. Grade as normal, decreased or absent.

SENSORY SYSTEM 6I

Have client close eyes for these tests; compare reactions for both sides of body.

1. Superficial tactile sensation — Compare sensitivity to wisp of cotton on each side of body; check hands, forearms, upper arms, trunk, thighs, lower legs, feet.

2. Superficial pain — Repeat procedure in 1, using sharp object.

3. Temperature — Repeat procedure in 1, testing ability to detect warm and cold by touching with test tube filled with water.

4. Sensitivity to vibration — Hold vibrating tuning fork to bony prominences: wrist, elbow, knee, ankle.

5. Joint position — Grasp digit between index finger and thumb, move passively and ask client to indicate direction of movement and final position of digit.

Continued

SENSORY SYSTEM—*Continued* 6J

6. *Two-point discrimination* — Using pins, lightly touch two parts of body close together simultaneously. Ask client if he is being touched by one or two points.

7. *Point localization* — With eyes closed, can client locate spot where touched?

8. *Stereognosis* — Can client recognize familiar objects such as apple, glass, pin by feeling them with hands while keeping eyes closed?

9. *Extinction phenomenon* — Touch two points simultaneously on opposite sides of the body in corresponding areas. With eyes closed, client should know that both sides were touched.

REFLEXES 6K

Deep Reflexes. Elicited by tapping briskly on a tendon or bony prominence, evoking sudden stretching of certain muscles and subsequent contraction.

Reflex	Site of Stimulus	Normal Response	Spinal Segment
Biceps	Biceps tendon	Contraction of biceps	C5, 6
Triceps	Triceps tendon above olecranon	Extension of elbow	C6, 7, 8
Brachioradialis	Lower third of radius	Flexion, pronation of forearm; flexion of fingers, hand	C5, 6
Patellar	Patellar tendon	Extension of leg at knee	L2, 3, 4
Achilles	Achilles tendon	Plantar flexion of foot	S1, 2
Plantar	Outer aspect of sole of foot	Plantar flexion of toes	S1, 2

Continued

REFLEXES—*Continued* 6L

Superficial Reflexes. Rapid firm stroking of skin with moderately sharp object, such as split tongue blade.

Reflex	Site of Stimulus	Normal Response	Spinal Segment
Abdominal	Stroke abdomen from periphery to umbilicus in 4 quads	Umbilicus moves toward area being stroked	T7, 8, 9
Cremasteric	Stroke inner aspects of thigh	Scrotum elevates	T12, L1

Abnormal Reflexes

Babinski — Stroking of lateral aspect of sole of foot causes dorsiflexion of big toe and fanning of toes.

Chaddock — Stroking of lateral aspect of foot beneath lateral malleolus causes same reflex as above.

Hoffmann — Extend client's wrists and third finger (at distal joint), flick fingertip up. Thumb flexes.

UNIT 12–HEAD AND NECK EXAMINATION 12A

GENERAL INSTRUCTIONS

1. Glasses are worn during acuity testing unless used only for reading.
2. If no Snellen chart available, have client read newspaper print at various distances.
3. If lesions are noted in mouth, palpate them with *gloved* hand; note characteristics.
4. Good lighting is essential.
5. Have all necessary equipment within reach.

HEALTH HISTORY: Ask client about 12B

1. History of injuries, medical Rx, surgery, dental problems, allergies, present medications, history of glaucoma or diabetes; wear glasses, hearing aid, dentures?
2. Smoking habits (packs/day or yr), exposure to loud noises, chemical irritants, geographical exposure.
3. Date of last visual/hearing test.
4. Current problems — Headaches, visual problems; earaches, hearing problems, ringing in ears, dizziness; sinus problems, runny nose, bleeding, sense of smell; soreness of mouth, tongue, gums, teeth, throat; difficulty swallowing, speech; swelling of neck lymph glands.

EYES 12C

1. Visual acuity — Client stands 20 ft from Snellen chart (one eye covered) and reads smallest print possible. Record result as feet away from chart/distance normal eye can read print line (e.g., 20/40 (mediated by II cranial nerve). Repeat with other eye.
2. Visual fields — Check client's ability to see hand movements in all 4 quadrants with one eye covered. Repeat with other eye.
3. External eye

General — State of face, expression, brows, blinking, position and alignment of eyes, prominence.

Lids — Height of palpebral fissure, depth of lids, edema, color, lesions, condition and direction of lashes.

Lacrimal ducts — Patency (press on nasal edge of lower lid — can express exudate if duct is blocked), excess tearing.

Conjunctiva — Color, growths; check lower and upper (upper, client looks down, grasp lashes and pull forward and down, place applicator stick across lid and push down to evert lid over stick. When client looks up, lid returns to normal position).

Continued

EYES—*Continued* 12D

Sclera — Note color.

Cornea and lens — Look from side with oblique lighting. Check depth of anterior chamber, curvature, opacities (shadows); should be shiny and bright.

Iris — Note color, consistency, borders.

Pupils — Check size, shape, equality. *Reaction to light*: direct (shine light into each pupil, observe constriction), consensual (observe simultaneous constriction when other pupil is directly constricted); *accommodation* (pupils dilate when focused on a far object, constrict when focused on finger held 6″ from nose).

4. *EOM's* — With head stationary, client follows examiner's hand through the six cardinal positions of gaze; pupils should move parallel without nystagmus or lid lag (mediated by III, IV, VI cranial nerves).

Convergence — Check ability of eyes to turn inward equally when looking at a close object.

Cover test for strabismus — Cover one eye, client looks straight ahead; remove cover and watch for movement of either eye; repeat on other side.

GENERAL INSTRUCTIONS: OPHTHALMOSCOPIC EXAM   12E

1. Semidark room to promote dilatation of pupils, prevent distracting reflections.

2. Check instrument for bright light; replace bulb and batteries if necessary.

3. Client and examiner seated, facing each other directly, heads at same level.

4. Both client and examiner remove glasses.

5. Ask client to focus on object straight ahead, not on ophthalmoscope light.

6. Use large white light for dilated pupils; small white light for constricted pupils.

7. Use right hand, right eye to examine right eye; use left hand, left eye to examine left eye.

OPACITIES   12F

1. Set lens at +6 diopters; approach directly from 4–6″.

2. Elicit red reflex — Move your head up, down, left, right; look for shadows (opacities).

To focus on opacity, use more positive setting than +6 if in lens, more negative than +6 if in cornea or deeper; determine apparent movement (opposite = corneal; stationary or movement in same direction = lens or deeper).

Note shape of opacity and location.

FUNDUSCOPY   12G

Approach client from 15° temporally until your foreheads touch. Reduce lens until the fundus is clear.

1. *Disc*

Observe shape (regular, irregular).

Observe margins — Distinct, indistinct, blurred. (If elevated, consider papilledema); crescents (pigment, sclera), myelinated nerve fibers at disc (congenital anomaly).

Color should be lighter and brighter pink than background (normal for disc to be darker nasally). Abnormal color (hyperemia = too red; optic atrophy = too pale).

Cup:disc ratio (diameter of cup to disc diameter) — Normal, less than 1:2(1:2 or greater is abnormal; suspect glaucoma).

2. *Vessels*

Observe distribution in all 4 quadrants; follow from disc to perimeter. Look for signs of occlusion: cherry red spot in macula, central retinal artery or vein hemorrhage, occlusion of branches (focal, plaque, edema).

Continued

FUNDUSCOPY—*Continued*   12H

Note caliber of vessels — Blood column smooth, regular decrease to periphery. Generalized narrowing, focal or multiple constrictions are abnormal.

AV ratio — 2:3 or 4:5 is normal; 1:2 or less is abnormal.

AV crossings — Insignificant unless blood flow interrupted (venous engorgement).

3. *General background*

Observe general retinal and choroidal pigmentation in relation to pigmentation of individual — Choroidal (fair-skinned persons), tigroid (dark-skinned persons).

Integrity of the retina — Examine for hemorrhages (solid = preretinal; linear or flame-shaped = superficial; dot or blot = deep); cotton-wool areas (cloud-like, obscure vessels); exudates (yellowish, flat, do not obscure vessels); drusen (normal in elderly persons; round, yellowish); retinal edema (milky appearance, obscures background); retinal detachment (periphery or gray fold).

4. Macula (approx. 2 disc diameters temporal from disc). Center (fovea) is very sensitive to light.

INTRAOCULAR PRESSURE   12I

Direct client to look downward with eyes closed. Use index fingers of both hands to apply gentle, alternating downward pressure to eyeball. Use one finger to press, one finger to assess movement and tension of eyeball. (Increased tension necessitates tonometric testing for glaucoma; decreased tension frequently due to dehydration.) Omit if there is eye pain, trauma or recent surgery!

USE OF THE OTOSCOPE

1. Select largest speculum that will fit into canal comfortably.
2. Client is seated with head tilted toward opposite shoulder.
3. Hold otoscope between thumb and first two fingers (not in palm) to avoid applying too much pressure.
4. With other hand, grasp pinna with thumb and fingers and pull out, up and back to straighten canal (out and down in children).
5. Insert speculum *slowly*, observing walls of canal and then tympanic membrane. Do *not* insert speculum *blindly*.

EARS   12J

1. External exam
Pinna — Look for deformity, lumps, lesions, tenderness.
Mastoid — Press firmly to detect tenderness.
2. Otoscopic exam
External canal — Look for wax, foreign bodies, discharge, redness, swelling, lesions.
Tympanic membrane — Note color, landmarks: malleus, umbo, light reflex, pars flaccida, pars tensa, anulus; bulging, retraction, scars, growths.
3. Auditory acuity
Distance client can hear spoken word or ticking watch (occlude one ear when testing, stand to side to avoid lip reading).
Weber test — Place vibrating tuning fork firmly on midline of scalp or forehead; client indicates where sound is loudest (should be equal in both ears).
Rinne test — Place vibrating fork firmly against mastoid process. When client can no longer hear it, hold fork in front of ear (do not restrike fork) until sound is no longer heard. Normal: Air conduction 2X greater than bone conduction.

NOSE   12K

1. *External* — Note deformities, asymmetry, inflammation, lesions.
2. *Internal* — Direct otoscope with nasal attachment posteriorly with head erect; tilt head back to see roof of cavity. *Nasal septum is sensitive!*
Patency: Look for foreign objects, polyps, tumors.
Mucosa: Check color, swelling, exudate, bleeding.
Septum: Look for bleeding, perforation, deviation.
Inferior and middle turbinates and middle meatus: Check color, swelling, exudate, polyps.
3. Palpate frontal and maxillary sinuses for tenderness.
4. Test sense of smell (mediated by I cranial nerve).

MOUTH AND PHARYNX   12L

1. Mouth
Lips — Check color, muscle, hydration, fissures, lesions, edema.
Buccal mucosa (use tongue blade and good lighting) — Note color, hydration, pigmentation, lesions, nodules.
Gums — Color, swelling, bleeding, lesions.
Teeth — Presence, shape, position, looseness, caries, repairs.
Gland ducts — Test for patency (check for calculi at openings of parotid glands in buccal mucosa opposite 2nd upper molar, and submaxillary openings from submaxillary glands at base of tongue).
Hard palate — Observe color, lesions, formation.
Tongue — On dorsum, note color, papillae, hydration, lesions. Have client stick tongue out, note size, shape, symmetry, lateral deviation and movement (test for strength, tremor, XII cranial nerve). On underside, look for white areas, nodules, ulcerations.

Continued

MOUTH AND PHARYNX—*Continued* 12M

2. Pharynx — Depress tongue in center with tongue blade; avoid touching uvula (causes gagging). Have client say "ah," watch for symmetrical rise of soft palate (uvula deviates to unaffected side if there is damage to X cranial nerve).

Check soft palate, ant. and post. pillars, uvula, tonsils, posterior pharynx for color, symmetry, exudate, edema, ulcer, enlargement.

3. Taste (tongue protruded, dry) — Test ant. 2/3 (VII cranial nerve) and post. 1/3 (IX cranial nerve); have client identify sweet, salt, bitter flavors of common items.

UNIT 13–EXAMINATION OF BREASTS AND AXILLAE 13A

GENERAL INSTRUCTIONS

1. Provide privacy (chaperone client according to agency policy).
2. Supply easily removable examining gown which covers upper body completely.
3. Examining room should be warm.
4. Anticipate that client may be anxious. Encourage client to discuss feelings; offer warm and reassuring attitude. Explain what you are doing *and why* throughout exam. If findings are *normal*, tell client.

NECK 12N

1. Inspect for symmetry, masses, scars.
2. Lymph nodes — Palpate with pads of fingers in rotating motion, client's head flexed slightly forward toward examiner. Note size, shape, delimitation, mobility, consistency and tenderness of any palpable node.

Preauricular nodes in front of ear.
Postauricular nodes anterior to mastoid process.
Occipital nodes, feel base of skull posteriorly.
Tonsillar nodes at angle of mandible.
Submaxillary nodes 1/2 way between angle and tip of mandible.
Submental nodes are midline beneath chin.
Superficial cervical nodes are superficial to sternomastoid.
Posterior cervical chain, anterior edge of trapezius.
Deep cervical chain, hook thumb and forefinger around sterno-cleidomastoid muscle.

Continued

NECK—*Continued* 12O

Supraclavicular, deep in angle formed by clavicle and sterno-cleidomastoid muscle.

3. Trachea — Inspect and palpate for deviation.
4. Identify hyoid bone, thyroid, cricoid cartilage.
5. Thyroid — Inspect for enlargement; palpate with client's neck flexed slightly forward and to one side; with one hand displace the thyroid cartilage to side, ask client to swallow, feel thyroid lateral lobe rise with fingers on other side; repeat for opposite side.
6. Strength of sternocleidomastoid and trapezius muscles — Have client shrug shoulders and turn head against resistance of examiner's hands (tests patency of XI cranial nerve).

HEALTH HISTORY: Ask client about

1. Any past Hx of breast lumps, surgeries (client or family), trauma; lactation, onset of menarche, last menstrual period, menopause.
2. Current problems — Lumps or changes in breasts, tenderness, rash, nipple discharge (color).
3. Medications — Contraceptives, pills, hormonal replacement during menopause?
4. Does client examine own breasts regularly? Has she been taught breast self-examination?
During examination, explain techniques of breast self-examination and supervise client's practice.

PALPATION

Breasts

1. Begin exam with client seated.
2. Apply palmar aspect of fingertips to outer quadrant of breasts; begin palpation with gentle rotary motion, moving toward nipple and then out.
3. If client complains of tenderness or lump in one breast, examine other breast first.
4. Systematically palpate entire breast (periphery, areola, tail) for *consistency* and *nodules* — Location, size, shape, consistency, delineation, mobility, tenderness.
5. Continue exam with client in supine position.
6. Place pillow under shoulder of side being examined to flatten breast tissue.
7. Repeat palpation, compressing breast tissue gently against chest wall.
8. Palpate nipple firmly, note elasticity, induration, subareolar masses; gently strip nipple to see whether discharge can be elicited (indicate amount and color).

Continued

INSPECTION

Client seated, arms and chest relaxed. All clothing removed to waist.

1. Breasts — Note size, symmetry.
Contour — Dimpling, masses, flattening
Skin — Color, thickening or edema, prominent venous pattern, rashes, scars.
2. Areolae and nipples — Size, shape, direction, bleeding, rashes, ulceration, discharge (color).
3. Inspect breast contours again for dimpling, retraction and symmetry while client raises arms over head; presses hands against hips to tense chest muscles. Have the client with large or pendulous breasts lean forward, supporting herself with hands on knees or on examiner's shoulders so that breasts hang free from chest wall.
4. Axillae and supraclavicular area — Support client's arm, sitting or supine. Observe for rashes, bulges, retractions, infections, edema.

PALPATION—Continued

Axillae

With client sitting or supine, support client's arm on side to be examined with your opposite hand.

1. Beginning with left side, cup examining fingers and reach high into apex of axilla.
2. Move fingers downward, exerting gentle pressure against ribs. Try to feel central nodes.
3. Repeat this movement inside ant. and post. axillary folds and against humerus. Try to feel pectoral, subscapular and lateral axillary nodes.
4. Repeat exam while arm is moved through full range of motion.
5. Examine right axilla using same technique.

Supraclavicular Area

Palpate for enlarged lymph nodes above and behind clavicle on both sides.
Note: Any suspicious breast findings must be checked by the physician immediately.

UNIT 16–RESPIRATORY EXAMINATION   16A

GENERAL INSTRUCTIONS

1. Examine client in *quiet* room.
2. Have client sit in relaxed position with shoulders drooping slightly forward.
3. Instruct client to breathe orally and slightly deeper than normal (increases intensity of breath sounds).
4. Systematically examine and compare each side of ant. and post. chest. Work down from apices.
5. Localize any abnormalities by intercostal space and distance from sternum, spine, midaxillary line, etc.

INSPECTION   16C

1. General
Position — Must client sit up to breathe?
Nutrition — Obesity may cause dyspnea.
Skin — Any cyanosis, excess veins, scar?
Nails — Clubbing?
Use of accessory respiratory muscles? Nasal flaring?
2. Chest — Skeletal deformities? Symmetry? AP diameter?
3. Respiratory rate — Regular or irregular? Depth?
4. Respiratory pattern
Women — Thoracic breathing, costal cage moves.
Men — Diaphragmatic, abdomen bulges.

HEALTH HISTORY: Ask client about   16B

1. Hx of TB (client or contacts), pneumonia, frequent colds, other lung disease.
2. Smoking habits (packs/day or yr), job hazards, geographical exposure.
3. Date of last chest x-ray, skin test.
4. Current problems, such as
Dyspnea — Exertional, paroxysmal, nocturnal, orthopnea.
Pain — Associated with breathing? Type, location, severity, duration, influencing factors.
Cough — Paroxysmal, effort-dependent, relation to position, productive.
Sputum — Color, odor, amount, time of day, hemoptysis.

PALPATION   16D

1. Check symmetry of expansion.
Stand behind client and place thumb of each hand just to side of spinal processes in midthoracic region. Extend tips of fingers to midaxillary lines on both sides. Have client inhale deeply. If asymmetry is present, one hand will be displaced further from midline than the other.
Place one hand on ant. chest and other hand on post. chest. Have client inhale deeply. Observe movement.
2. Palpate each rib and all portions of chest wall with firm pressure. Any pain or discomfort?
3. Note position of trachea — Place index finger firmly into supra-sternal notch and locate tracheal rings in relation to sternum. A shift indicates shift in mediastinal structures.
4. Tactile fremitus — With client seated, have him repeat "ninety-nine" in a deep voice. Move your hands on chest from apices to bases. Compare intensity and symmetry of vibrations.

PERCUSSION 16E

1. Patient may be sitting or standing. Percuss downward from apices; first front, then back. Strike with equal force on left and right sides of chest and compare degree of resonance.

2. Determine diaphragmatic excursion

Ask client to inhale deeply and hold breath.

Percuss downward from apices until normal resonance changes to dull. Mark with a line.

Instruct client to exhale completely and hold breath. Percuss down and mark point of transition from resonance to dullness.

Normal excursion is 3–6 cm.

AUSCULTATION 16F

Use diaphragm of stethoscope. Listen to back, alternating left and right parallel points, moving from apices to bases. Repeat on front.

1. Concentrate on *quality* of breath sounds.
2. Compare length of inspiration with length of expiration.
3. Listen for abnormal breath sounds — Absent, diminished, friction rubs, bronchial, bronchovesicular.
4. Listen for adventitious breath sounds — Rales, rhonchi, wheezes. Do they disappear after coughing?
5. If consolidation or compression of lung tissue is suspected, auscultate for abnormal voice sounds.

Bronchophony — Client repeats "99" (syllables audible).

Egophony — Client repeats "E" (heard as "A").

Whispered pectoriloquy — Client whispers "99" (whispered word clearly perceived through stethoscope).

UNIT 20–CARDIOVASCULAR EXAMINATION 20A

GENERAL INFORMATION

1. Examine in good light in quiet room.
2. Patient should be on firm surface, both sitting and recumbent.
3. All clothing removed from chest. Towel may be used to drape female breasts.
4. Examination of woman with large breasts accomplished by holding breast upward and to the left. Client may do this.
5. Findings should be described in relation to cardiac cycle (systolic, diastolic, presystolic) and location on precordium (i.e., 3rd intercostal space 4 cm from midsternal line).

HEALTH HISTORY: Ask client about 20B

1. Chief complaint — "What has been bothering you?"
2. Past Hx — Early cardiac murmur, rheumatic fever; venereal disease and Rx; injuries, pregnancies, medications, surgeries.
3. Current Hx — Pain (type, location, duration, precipitating causes), dyspnea, orthopnea, PND, fatigue, edema, palpitations, fainting, cyanosis? Allergies, medications.
4. Social Hx — Occupations, hobbies, unusual life patterns.
5. Habits — Drugs, alcohol, tobacco.
6. Family Hx — Heart disease (congenital, acute, chronic), hypertension, diabetes mellitus, arteriosclerosis; CVA.

1. Client in supine position or with head and chest slightly elevated.
2. Compare chest for symmetry.
3. Locate lines of reference (midsternal, midclavicular) and identify intercostal spaces.
4. Visually locate apical area, tricuspid area, Erb's point, pulmonary area, aortic area, epigastric area.
5. Observe thoracic configuration — Barrel chest, bulges, pectus carinatum, pectus excavatum.
6. Note nutritional status — Thin, obese, emaciated.
7. Respirations — Rate, rhythm, dyspnea.
8. Skin — Color changes? Note vascularity.
9. Stand to client's right and use tangential lighting to note any precordial pulsations.
10. Identify PMI — Note location, amplitude, size (apical beat not always observable).

1. Stand to client's right and place right palm over apical area.
2. Locate apical beat with index or middle finger. Note location, amplitude, duration, size; observe rate, rhythm, presence of any thrills.
3. If you have difficulty locating apical pulse, have client turn to left lateral position and exhale. This maneuver will bring apex closer to chest wall; however, it should not be used to identify location since it displaces apex to left.
4. Clients with thick chest walls or emphysema should be put in sitting position and asked to lean slightly forward during palpation.
5. Move palm over tricuspid area, Erb's point, pulmonary area, aortic area (observe any pulsations, thrills, vibrations).

1. With client supine, stand at right and apply diaphragm of stethoscope to apical area.
2. Listen closely and identify first and second heart sounds (S_1 and S_2).

S_1 is first of the paired heart sounds. It is deeper and longer than S_2.

If heart rate is rapid, place a finger over PMI while listening. S_1 will be synchronous with rise of finger. Carotid pulse may also be used to time S_1. It occurs immediately after S_1.

3. Continue to listen until you have correctly identified the two heart sounds.
4. Diagram intensity and duration of S_1 and S_2 at apical area.
5. Count heart rate; identify rhythm as regular, irregular, regularly irregular.
6. Place bell of stethoscope lightly on apical area — listen for abnormal heart sounds (S_3 and S_4); turn client to left lateral position, listen again for S_3 and S_4.

Continued

7. Return client to supine position and after again identifying S_1 and S_2 begin to slowly inch stethoscope toward tricuspid area (use diaphragm).
8. Inch along left sternal border to Erb's point.
Note intensity of S_1 and S_2.
Have client inhale, note any physiological splitting of S_2.
Continue to listen as client exhales; does splitting disappear?
9. Inch stethoscope up to pulmonary area and then across to aortic area (base of heart).
Compare intensity of sounds at pulmonary area and aortic area.
Note intensity of S_1 and S_2 in this area; diagram and compare with intensity and duration of sounds at apical area.
10. Have client sit up. Listen at each auscultatory area again with both diaphragm and bell.
11. Listen for abnormal sounds — Sounds preceding S_2 are systolic; those after S_2 are diastolic.
12. Listen for murmurs — Describe timing in cardiac cycle, location, radiation (if any), intensity (grades I through VI), pitch, quality.

UNIT 21–ABDOMINAL EXAMINATION 21A

GENERAL INFORMATION

1. Client relaxed, supine with arms at sides, knees flexed with feet flat on table. Room should be warm. Client is draped from nipples up, pubis down; cold tends to increase peristalsis. Have client empty bladder before examination.

2. Examination is performed from client's right side; tangential lighting aids observation of pulsations; auscultation is performed before palpation or percussion, since the latter maneuvers tend to distort normal abdominal sounds. Each quadrant is systematically examined, leaving tender areas for last.

3. Masses and hernias are best observed when client is standing, due to pressure on organs and pull of gravity.

INSPECTION 21C

1. *Position of comfort* — Leaning forward, lying still and rigid, writhing.
2. *Abdominal contour* — Protuberant, obese, scaphoid.
3. *Symmetry* — Asymmetry due to fluid, air, tumor, hernia, pregnancy.
4. *Skin* — Color, lesions, vessel pattern, scars.
5. *Umbilicus* — Direction, contour, hernia, lesions.
6. *Movements* — Peristalsis, pulsations (aneurysm, abnormal blood flow).

HEALTH HISTORY: Ask client about 21B

1. *Past Hx* of illness, surgery or trauma involving appendix, gallbladder, spleen, liver, GI tract, GU tract; hernias, hepatitis.
2. Medications, diet, alcohol, prosthesis (colostomy, IUD, truss).
3. *Current problems* — Abdominal pain (location, quality, onset, aggravating/alleviating factors, associated Sx's), malaise, anorexia, nausea, vomiting, wt. loss or gain, fever, diarrhea, constipation, melena, jaundice, cloudy or burning urine.

AUSCULTATION 21D

Warm stethoscope, light pressure; listen for 2–3 min in each quadrant and over epigastrium.

1. *Bowel sounds* — Absent (paralytic ileus), increased (gastritis, early obstruction), gurgling/tinkling (late obstruction before ileus), borborygmi (stomach growling). Bowel sounds heard best just below and to the right of umbilicus.
2. *Circulatory sounds* — Bruits (abnormal blood flow in aorta, femoral arteries), venous hums (AV fistulas over organs), rubs (peritoneal irritation).

LIGHT PALPATION 21E

Use light, firm pressure; avoid tickling.
1. *Muscular tension* — Rigidity (involuntary), guarding (voluntary).
2. *Enlarged organ* — Pregnant uterus, other.
3. *Masses* — Indicate location and approximate size.

DEEP PALPATION

Use two hands, one on top of other.
1. *Masses* — Location, shape, consistency, tenderness, pulsations, mobility.
2. *Rebound tenderness* over tender areas — press slowly, withdraw fingers quickly — if there is peritoneal involvement, client will have rebound pain when hand withdrawn.
3. *Liver* — With left hand push up from back under 11th–12th ribs; starting at iliac crest; with right hand, press in (firmly) and up toward the costal margin. Feel liver hit fingertips during deep inspiration. Normal = 1–2 cm below costal margin. Edge should be sharp, straight, without nodules.
Continued

UNIT 22–GENITOURINARY AND RECTAL EXAMINATION (MALE) 22A

GENERAL INFORMATION

1. Provide appropriate drape as necessary and privacy from interruption. Maintain professional approach and respect for client's concerns.
2. Examiner must have short fingernails to prevent discomfort.
3. Client may sit on edge of exam table or be supine for inspection and palpation of the genitals. Client standing, with examiner seated, is recommended for assessment of hernias. Rectal exam may be performed with the client in (1) left lateral position or (2) standing, leaning over table.
4. Gloves are recommended for palpation and are mandatory for examining any lesions or discharge. Obtain specimens of any discharge. Urine sample helpful in differentiating some GU problems.

DEEP PALPATION—*Continued* 21F

4. *Spleen* (not usually palpated unless greatly enlarged) — Standing at client's right, reach across abdomen and pull left lower rib cage up with left hand. Press deeply with right hand toward spleen, under costal margin. Record cm below costal margin.
5. *Kidneys* — Most easily felt in persons with relaxed abdominal walls. Right kidney lower than left. Support right flank (below 12th rib) with left hand; press *very* deeply with right hand in *lower* right quadrant; feel lower pole of kidney come down to your fingertips during deep inspiration. Palpate left kidney in same manner; stand to client's right, as in palpating spleen.
6. *CVA* (costovertebral angle) *tenderness* — Hit fist against flat hand along posterior CV margin (kidney infection) and anterior margin (liver, splenic inflammation).
7. *Aorta* — Use one or two hands, press fingertips on either side of aorta, deep in upper abdomen, to left of midline. Note whether pulsations are increased, transmitted forward (normal) or lateral (abnormal).

PERCUSSION 21G

1. Note *gas pattern* in abdomen; general areas of dullness; tympany over gastric bubble — Percuss left ant. axillary line, 10th ICS.
2. *Liver* — To check size, percuss in right midclavicular line from level of resonance below umbilicus upward to liver dullness (approx. at costal margin); percuss along same line downward from lung resonance to liver dullness (approx. 7th ICS). Normal size, 6–12 cm, females smaller than males. If enlargement suspected, percuss for size again, in midsternal line. Borders may be obscured by gas in colon or fluid in lungs.
3. *Spleen* — Percuss lowest interspace in left ant. axillary line. If spleen is *not* enlarged, sound is tympanic or resonant due to gastric air (sometimes splenic dullness can be percussed posterior to left axillary line in 10th ICS).
4. *Bladder* — Percuss dullness of distended bladder.
5. *Masses* — Percuss borders to estimate size.
6. *Fluid levels* — In shifting dullness, fluid flows with gravity, air rises. If large amounts of ascitic fluid suspected, have client turn on side; percussion over fluid is dull, over air, resonant.

HEALTH HISTORY: Ask client about   22B

1. Hx of surgery (circumcision, hernia, hemorrhoids, prostate), trauma, urinary tract infections, venereal disease, carcinoma (client or family).

2. Current medications, other illnesses (cardiac, renal), prosthesis (truss).

3. Current problems — Discharge or lesions, difficult or frequent urination; testicular tenderness, change in size; hernia; constipation, hemorrhoids, rectal bleeding; sexual difficulties; pain.

PENIS

1. Observe distribution of pubic hair; size, shape, skin color, lesions, edema, nodules.

2. Ask client to retract prepuce; observe glans for hygiene (accumulation of smegma), size and placement of urethral meatus, discharge, lesions. Palpate (with gloves) for induration, tenderness; palpate shaft for nodules, plaques, tenderness.

SCROTUM   22C

1. Inspect general size, contour, skin color.

2. Spread walls of scrotum between your fingers. Note any lesions, nodules. Lift to inspect posterior surface. Compare contents of both sides simultaneously using thumbs and forefingers; identify oval *testes;* note size, shape, tenderness, consistency, nodules, symmetry.

3. Identify comma-shaped *epididymides* on posterior surface of testes; check symmetry, tenderness, size.

4. Identify spermatic cords simultaneously — Grasp cord on each side, at neck of scrotum, between thumb and forefinger. Gently palpate length down to testes. Vas deferens felt as single, hard cord surrounded by less distinct strands (blood vessels, etc.). Note any masses or thickening.

5. Transilluminate any abnormal swelling. Hold penlight behind each side of the scrotum. Structures containing serous fluid transmit light as a red glow. Blood and tissue block passage of light.

GROIN   22D

Client standing with examiner seated in front.

1. Inspect inguinal and femoral regions for scars, lesions, enlarged lymph nodes, hernia bulges. Ask client to strain or bear down to accentuate bulges (indirect hernia most commonly seen in middle of inguinal area; direct hernia is nearer to symphysis; femoral hernia is below inguinal ligament near symphysis).

2. Palpate inguinal canal — Starting at lower end of scrotal sac, invaginate loose folds as you direct your finger tip up into external inguinal ring. Ask client to cough: indirect hernia will tap against fingertip; if direct hernia, impulse is felt through posterior canal wall. Note that indirect hernias frequently pass on into scrotum and must be differentiated from other scrotal masses.

RECTUM   22E

Client standing, leaning over table; or in left lateral position with right knee drawn up to chest.

1. Before starting, let client know that procedure will make him feel as if he were moving his bowels and that he should not be alarmed.

2. Glove examining hand. Squirt lubricant onto paper towel for easy access (avoid excess). Readjust exam light as necessary.

3. Inspect sacrococcygeal and perianal areas for inflammation, lesions. Spread buttocks with nonexamining hand and inspect anal area.

4. Lubricate tip of gloved index finger, ask client to strain or bear down — note hemorrhoids. Place tip of finger over anus. As client relaxes, finger inserts easily past rectal sphincter. Direct exam finger toward umbilicus, noting any laxity or abnormal tightness of sphincter.

5. Palpate right lateral, posterior and left lateral walls of rectum. Turn your hand to examine anterior surface: identify two lobes of prostate gland and note size, shape, consistency, nodularity or tenderness. Feel above prostate if possible.

6. Withdraw finger gently. Test any fecal material on glove for occult blood. Give client tissues for wiping.

GENERAL INFORMATION

1. Relaxation is essential for comfort of client and adequate examination. Ask client to empty bladder; obtain urine specimen if needed.

2. All clothing is removed (only from waist down if breast exam not being done). Shoes may be worn if stirrups are not padded.

3. Assist client into lithotomy position with buttocks slightly extended over end of table. Thighs flexed and comfortably abducted. Support head with small pillow (helps to relax abdominal muscles). Drape properly — one drape over chest and a square drape over abdomen and knees with one corner between the legs (folded back during examination).

4. Have all equipment at hand including good lighting, vaginal speculum of appropriate size. (Before use, speculum is warmed and lubricated with water. Test temperature of blades before inserting. Do not use any other lubricant if you are obtaining specimens.)

Continued

GENERAL INFORMATION—*Continued*
23B

5. (Use lubricant sparingly; spread a small amount on blades with your finger.) *Note:* Gloves are always changed if vagina is examined after rectum. It is advisable to change gloves between vaginal and rectal exams to prevent possible spread of gonorrhea to rectum; blood cells from vagina will give false positive result when checking rectally for occult blood.

6. Examiner is seated at foot of table. Maintain verbal contact to assess client's reactions. Explain purpose and steps in procedures before performing them.

7. Male examiners traditionally have female attendant.

HEALTH HISTORY: Ask client about

1. Surgery (C-section, hysterectomy), injury, illness (VD, kidney disease, urinary tract infection), blood clots, familial Hx of cancer.

2. Menstrual Hx (menarche age, climacteric age, postmenopausal bleeding), last menstrual period, characteristics of flows; OB history (para, gravida, abortions).

EXTERNAL GENITALIA
23C

1. Inspect mons pubis, labia majora, perineum. Note distribution of pubic hair, inflammation, swelling, lesions, growths, scars.

2. Separate labia and inspect vestibule. Note inflammation, swelling, lesions, discharge, atrophy, abnormal odor. Examine the following:

Labia minora.

Clitoris — Size varies; endocrine disorders and medications may cause enlargement.

Urethral opening — Skene's glands located below opening, not readily visible (with inflammation obtain specimen by milking urethra with index finger outward); caruncle; prolapse of urethral mucosa in meatus.

Vaginal introitus — Check Bartholin's glands. Palpate tissue on each side between thumb, on outside of labia and index finger, in vagina; culture any discharge. Record presence or absence of hymen.

3. Assess strength of perineal muscles — Spread labia with gloved index and middle fingers of right hand, ask client to strain or bear down. Bulging of ant. vaginal wall (cystocele) or posterior wall and rectum (rectocele).

INTERNAL GENITALIA
23D

1. Select speculum; check to see that blades are aligned and firmly closed.

2. Place first two fingers of your right hand (left hand if left handed) at vaginal introitus and press down on perineum. With left hand insert closed speculum with blades at 45° angle over your fingers. Direct speculum downward to avoid sensitive anterior wall of vagina and urethra. Remove right hand and turn blades into horizontal position.

3. While continuing to exert downward pressure, open blades and visualize cervical os. Tighten thumb screw to keep blades in position.

Size and position of os (points upward if uterus is retroverted) — In nulliparous women, os is usually small round or oval opening; in parous women, os is slitlike. Also note string from intrauterine device (IUD) if present.

Color — Inflammation with vaginitis; bluish color with pregnancy, neoplasm, congestive heart failure (cyanosis).

Continued

INTERNAL GENITALIA—*Continued*   23E

Lesions — Neoplasm, venereal disease, lacerations from childbirth (unilateral or bilateral transverse; stellate), erosions.

Masses — Bright red polyps, translucent cysts, carcinoma.

Discharge or bleeding.

4. Cytological specimens (Papanicolaou smears); obtain in following order and fix immediately.

Endocervical swab — Rotate cotton-tipped swab moistened with saline in os. Swab across glass slide gently.

Ectocervical scrape — Place long end of spatula in os; rotate with firm pressure; smear on second slide. (If cervix has been removed, scrape vaginal cuff.)

Vaginal pool — Roll cotton-tipped swab on vaginal floor below cervix; smear on third slide.

5. *Vaginal walls* — Note color, lesions, masses.

6. Slowly withdraw speculum with left hand. After blades clear cervix, release thumb screw while keeping blades in open position with thumb. Assess walls of vagina as speculum is withdrawn. Close blades completely as passing introitus.

BIMANUAL EXAMINATION (Examiner standing)   23F

1. Lubricate first two fingers of gloved right hand and insert in downward position into vagina, keeping thumb abducted and other fingers flexed. Palpate walls for growths or tenderness. (Use only one finger if introitus is very small.)

2. Cervix — Note position, shape, consistency, mobility, tenderness (normally feels firm like the tip of your nose, smooth, mobile and nontender). Softening of cervix with pregnancy = Hegar's sign.

3. Palpate fornix surrounding cervix, note nodules.

4. Uterus — Note size, shape, position, consistency, mobility, tenderness.

With left hand (right hand if left-handed), press downward in midline of abdomen; with right hand press straight inward and upward under cervix to trap uterus between fingers of both hands. (It is helpful to support your forearm on a raised knee or hip.) Assess characteristics of uterus between your two hands; normally firm, smooth, mobile, nontender.

Continued

BIMANUAL EXAMINATION (Examiner standing)—*Continued*   23G

Move your abdominal hand to left and right lower quadrants as pelvic fingers move to left and right lateral fornices. Assess left and right ovaries for tenderness or enlargement. (Normally ovary is not palpable but slightly tender.) If present, identify size, shape, mobility, tenderness, any adnexal masses.

5. Rectovaginal exam — Alert client that this procedure will make her feel as if she needs to have a bowel movement. Withdraw your fingers from vagina and change gloves. Lubricate first two fingers. Reintroduce index finger into vagina while inserting middle finger into rectum. Exert pressure with abdominal hand as before. In this procedure the rectal finger palpates behind cervix and posterior surface of uterus.

RECTAL EXAMINATION   23H

1. During preceding maneuver, palpate rectal wall for masses, tenderness; note sphincter tone. Test fecal material adhering to glove for occult blood. Don't forget to inspect perianal area for inflammation, lesions, nodules.

2. Assist client out of stirrups and provide tissues for wiping.